A Clinical Guide to Autistic Spectrum Disorders

Patricia Evans, M

Associate Professor of Neur
Pediatrics Director
Neurodevelopmental Disabi
University of Texas Southwe
Dallas, Texas

Mary Ann Morri:

Coordinator Psychometrici
Neurology Department
Children's Medical Center
Dallas, Texas

Wolters Kluwer | Lipp
Health
Philadelphia • Baltimore • New York • L
Buenos Aires • Hong Kong • Sydney • Tc

Acquisitions Editor: Sonya Seigafuse
Product Manager: Nicole Walz
Vendor Manager: Bridgett Dougherty
Senior Manufacturing Manager: Benjamin Rivera
Marketing Manager: Lisa Lawrence
Design Coordinator: Stephen Druding
Production Service: Aptara, Inc.

Printed in China

Library of Congress Cataloging-in-Publication Data
Evans, Patricia, 1956- author.
   A clinical guide to autistic spectrum disorders / Patricia Evans, MD, FAAN, FAAP, Associate Professor of Neurology, Pediatrics Director, Neurodevelopmental Disabilities Residency, University of Texas Southwestern School of Medicine, Dallas, Texas, Mary Ann Morris, PhD, Coordinator Psychometrician, Neurology Department, Children's Medical Center of Dallas, Dallas, Texas.
      p. ; cm.
   Includes bibliographical references and index.
   ISBN 978-1-60831-269-6 (pbk. : alk. paper) 1. Autism spectrum disorders. 2. Autism in children. 3. Autism spectrum disorders—Treatment. I. Morris, Mary Ann, author. II. Title.
   [DNLM: 1. Child Development Disorders, Pervasive—diagnosis. 2. Child Development Disorders, Pervasive—therapy. WS 350.6]
   RC553.A88E945 2011
   618.92'85882—dc22   2010046744

Care has been taken to confirm the accuracy of the information presented and to describe generally accepted practices. However, the authors, editors, and publisher are not responsible for errors or omissions or for any consequences from application of the information in this book and make no warranty, expressed or implied, with respect to the currency, completeness, or accuracy of the contents of the publication. Application of the information in a particular situation remains the professional responsibility of the practitioner.

   The authors, editors, and publisher have exerted every effort to ensure that drug selection and dosage set forth in this text are in accordance with current recommendations and practice at the time of publication. However, in view of ongoing research, changes in government regulations, and the constant flow of information relating to drug therapy and drug reactions, the reader is urged to check the package insert for each drug for any change in indications and dosage and for added warnings and precautions. This is particularly important when the recommended agent is a new or infrequently employed drug.

   Some drugs and medical devices presented in the publication have Food and Drug Administration (FDA) clearance for limited use in restricted research settings. It is the responsibility of the health care provider to ascertain the FDA status of each drug or device planned for use in their clinical practice.

To purchase additional copies of this book, call our customer service department at (800) 638-3030 or fax orders to (301) 223-2320. International customers should call (301) 223-2300.

Visit Lippincott Williams & Wilkins on the Internet: at LWW.com. Lippincott Williams & Wilkins customer service representatives are available from 8:30 am to 6 pm, EST.

10 9 8 7 6 5 4 3 2 1

CCS0111

To Lana

PREFACE

In the mid-1980s, I had the great good fortune to practice alongside two gentlemen who were truly pediatricians of the "old school." Both men trained in the 1950s, prior to the creation of many of the vaccines routinely used now, to say nothing of the range of sophisticated antimicrobials and other pharmaceuticals now available in the early 21st century. Dr. T.H. Holmes Jr. and the late Dr. Gene Rankin remain my earliest and best mentors for the practice of medicine, not only for their vast expertise of children's illnesses but also because of their capacity for practicing exceptionally high standard of care in all aspects of their practice. This standard was all the more striking because of the incredible volume of patients and virtual absence of subspecialists within hundreds of miles of their base in Lubbock, Texas. A typical day for each of these gentlemen was to start morning rounds on their in-patient service and several newborns before 8 AM; stop and have breakfast in the hospital doctor's lounge; go on to see 60 or more both sick and well children over the course of the next 10 hours; make evening rounds; then rotate a 1 in 2 call schedule to handle after hour emergency phone calls, whether real or perceived on the part of the parent. Both men worked at this intensity for literally decades. Subsequently, it was my great privilege to have been part of that team for a few brief years.

After 5 years of practicing alongside these giants of primary care pediatrics, I pursued additional training to better understand neurodevelopmental disorders in children. But I have never forgotten the unrelenting hard physical and emotional work it took to be a primary care pediatrician. I continue to have great appreciation for both of these gentlemen, and am so grateful for the teaching they provided me. Both men profoundly influenced my understanding of children and their families.

To that end, this text is written in honor of Dr. Holmes and Dr. Rankin, as well as all pediatric practitioners who work tirelessly to serve children and their families. There are many excellent, reflective, and important texts available about autism available, and I have tried to list only a representative few at the end of this text. However, this small handbook is specifically designed to help primary care providers, including pediatricians, family practitioners, internists, and nurse practitioners, move as efficiently as possible through the day. The handouts to families, potential letters to teachers, and suggestions on creating an autism team that costs the practitioner nothing, as well as a fairly extensive flow chart for the myriad of symptoms, are all offered to maximize the few minutes available in each physician—family interview. My hope is that these are particularly helpful, when in the context of either a well or sick visit, the parents ask about worrisome complaints (often when a child is having her ears examined!) about odd behaviors, exceptional rages, delays that were not noticed just 3 months ago at the last visit, and even just academic and social issues that are odd or worrisome. Primary care providers are busy: between writing the scripts for acute illness and attempting to assess how serious the behavioral complaints are, this text with its charts and forms is offered as one way to streamline complex symptoms.

Section I is a topical introduction to autism and includes salient points of history of our understanding of the disorder.

Section II consists of brief chapters that are organized by presenting symptoms. The first chapter of this section contains a pull-out composite flow chart for use in lab coat pockets, if desired, as well as a suggestion for building an "autism team" of professionals that can be particularly helpful for the primary care physician to consider as a way of streamlining care. The chapters that follow then are grouped by symptoms with a sample case for each chapter, followed by a brief discussion, followed by its flow chart, taken, respectively, from the composite flow chart at the beginning of the section. Special mention is made of individuals who may be exceptionally prodigious in some areas, the rare individual with an autistic savant diagnosis, who may be gifted in music or rapid math calculations, but quite impaired with socialization or communication. An additional chapter is provided exploring ways to specifically assist adults living with varying degrees of ASDs and for whom public school services are not available, adequate, or appropriate. Finally, a brief word regarding potential ethical concerns is included, specific to the need to consider inclusivity as much as possible, autonomy when able, and dignity for the person always.

Section III deals with therapeutic aspects of autism, specifically environmental suggestions, nonmedication therapeutics, and medication approaches. An additional chapter reviews controversial alternative autism treatments, which is based on lack of peer-reviewed data, should be avoided.

Section IV speaks to current U.S. federal public education law regarding the needs of children with autistic spectrum disorder. Included in this section are autism assessment guidelines for the medical and school settings, sample medical statements that the primary care physician is encouraged to generate with his or her own professional logo, if helpful. A final brief statement deals with advocacy, and the enormous power of the prescription pad, even in a 5-minute patient visit, and how best to advocate for your patient and his or her family in a fast and effective manner.

Finally, appendices are provided both in print as well as in the accompanying CD, which permits easy printing of any of the suggested Autism Spectrum Questionnaires, Behavior Diaries for Families, and Autism Spectrum Handouts that are age and symptoms based. Finally, handouts for families on how to best interact with public school are also provided.

References are also provided for the physician who wishes a more thorough discussion on the neurobiology and research approaches that are currently underway. A subject index is also provided for ready reference to contents of the handbook.

It's been nearly 30 years since, as a pediatrician, I charged $25 a child, and pediatricians routinely asked parents to bill their own insurance. With the advent of managed care and electronic record keeping, quite apart from the sheer volume of medical expertise needed to treat children, primary care medicine is far more complex. However, what hasn't changed is that we still are restricted to not more than 24 hours in a day, and just as many children need our on-going energetic care and advocacy. This text is respectfully offered to this front line of dedicated individuals, specifically primary care physicians, nurses, educators, and social workers, with the hope that the information, charts, chapters, and appendices will be of help in their day-to-day work of caring for children.

Patricia Evans, MD
May, 30th, 2010
Frisco, Texas

ACKNOWLEDGMENTS

I would like to particularly express my thanks to the following individuals:

To Dr. Susan Iannaccone, whose unflagging support and shared vision of what a neurodevelopmental disabilities program could be, has helped create the current Neurodevelopmental Disabilities Program at the University of Texas Southwestern School of Medicine, Division of Child Neurology; with the stated mission of creating a program that provides excellent care to all children regardless of capacity to pay.

To Dr. Mary Ann Morris, for her wisdom and expertise in the psychological assessment of these wonderful but often puzzling children, as well as her passion for advocacy for all children to be seen and served.

To Reverend Ted Dotts, who from the beginning taught me and so many others what it means to practice inclusivity and advocacy.

To Dr. Steve Roach, for the exceptional mentoring as my former child neurology fellowship chair and his on-going support as well, particularly with regard to the literary process.

To Dr. Roger Brumback, for his helpful suggestions and edits and for his championing of our shared concern about the epic rise of unsafe and undocumented treatments particularly in the context of autism.

To Nicole Walz, at Lippincott Williams & Wilkins, whose patience and guidance was so generously offered in the creation of this text.

To my late older sister, Lana Evans Maney, and her commitment to be authentically herself in spite of many challenges and hardships along the way; and to our mother, Charlotte Evans Ayers, who relentlessly advocated for her needs.

And, most importantly, to my husband Johnny, who supported me every step of the way, and whose excellent suggestions and commentary regarding both form and content were indispensable.

P.A.E.

I would like to take the opportunity to recognize and honor the people who have supported me in my efforts. Words cannot fully express the gratitude I have for my parents, Oliver and Marilyn Sturrock, who encouraged life-long learning and demonstrated that worthwhile endeavors take dedication, determination, and hard work. I would like to especially thank my son, Riley, my family, and my friends for their incredible love and untiring support. I deeply appreciate my friend and colleague Dr. Patricia Evans for her incredible knowledge about the special needs population, as well as her guidance, thoughtful insights, and support.

M.A.M.

CONTENTS

Appendices

Section One:

Introduction to Autistic Spectrum Disorders

History

Individuals with features of autism have been described in literature long before this century. In 1911 the brilliant Swiss psychiatrist Eugen Bleuler (1857–1939) was the first to use the term "autism" in a medical setting (1–6). As the director of a hospital in Zurich, Bleuler created the word *autism* along with *schizophrenia*, and *ambivalence*. Autism stems from the Greek word *autos* meaning self. Bleuler's description of autism referred to a form of schizophrenia in which the individual was extremely withdrawn from the outside world into the self. Rather than a separate condition, Bleuler's "autism" was thought to be a basic problem seen in schizophrenia of all ages.

Bleuler's description of an individual with autism included detachment from reality and enmeshed with a rich fantasy life or delusional thinking that he referred to as an inner life. This inner-life component has been dispelled along with several other descriptors (e.g., deranged hierarchy of values and goals); however, he did include in the clinical description of autism poor ability to interact with others and the display of inappropriate behaviors that have continued to be components of the diagnosis of autism today.

In 1943 Dr. Leo Kanner (1894–1981), a child psychiatrist at Johns Hopkins University, was the first to describe autism as a specific disorder in a clinical context. He based his discovery on 11 children he observed between 1938 and 1943. He studied children who had withdrawn from human contact as early as 1 year of age. His article "Autistic Disturbances of Affective Contact" described characteristics shared by these children as "extreme autistic aloneness" as well as total indifference to other people that began at the very beginning of life. Kanner introduced the term "early infantile autism," which has also been called Kanner's syndrome. His use of Bleuler's term suggests that he believed these children were trying to escape from reality. His decision to use the term may have inadvertently contributed to views that autism was a psychologically based disorder rather than being biological in nature.

The year after Kanner published his article, an Austrian scientist and pediatrician Hans Asperger (1906–1980) published "Autistic Psychopathy in Childhood." The case study was of children who presented with recognizable and similar characteristics that he came to call autistic psychopaths. Nevertheless, because the article was not available in English, Asperger's work would not be widely known until 40 years later in 1981.

Kanner and Bleuler both used the term autism and both noted that this type of disturbance appeared to have been present from birth. They also noted a common feature of an inability to develop and maintain normal interpersonal relationships. In addition, Asperger noted that the children in his study all had speech and spoke like *little grownups*, as well as exhibited clumsy motor skills. Asperger's disorder was not officially recognized as a form of autism until 1994.

In Kanner's 1943 article he noted that there appeared to be a lack of warmth among the parents of children with autism. Subsequently, much was written about this perceived lack of affection shown to the children by their parents. In 1949 Kanner wrote a paper that suggested that children with autism appeared to withdraw in order to seek comfort in themselves because of a lack of maternal warmth and distant fathers.

During the 1950s, the term "refrigerator mother" grew from this supposition with the assistance of the Freudian-based psychoanalytic view that a child could not progress if basic psychological bonds were not formed early in life. This theory dismissed alternative theories that the parents' presumed emotionally distant behavior could be a response to lack of reciprocation of affection from their child or that the characteristics seen in the children could be genetically inherited traits.

Dr. Bruno Bettelheim (1903–1990), a controversial Austrian-American child psychologist, wrote *The Empty Fortress: Infantile Autism and the Birth of the Self* in 1967. He wrote that the underlying cause of autism was unresponsive parents who were unable to bond with their child. Bettelheim's studies and writings perpetuated the theory initiated by Kanner of *refrigerator mothers* and inadequate parenting that continued through the 1970s and likely beyond (7).

DEFINITION

Autism is a neurological and developmental disorder characterized by distinctive impairments in social interaction, communication (verbal and nonverbal), and unusual behaviors and interests. Approximately 70% of individuals with autism also have mental retardation and it is four times more common in men than in women (8,9).

Children with autism exhibit an atypical developmental pattern. Indications of problems may be apparent at birth, but difficulties most often become more evident as a child progresses in age. Some children attain developmental milestones at the expected time, but between 12 and 36 months of age begin to regress. There can be changes in behaviors and reactions to people, as well as regression of communication, social, and/or other previously attained skills. This may be a sudden onset or occur at a slower rate.

Autism (also referred to as autistic disorder) is one of five disorders that fall under the umbrella term of pervasive developmental disorders (PDDs) of the *Diagnostic and Statistical Manual of Mental Disorders—Fourth Edition Text Revision (DSM–IV–TR)* (Table 1.1) (10). The term PDD is frequently referred to as autistic spectrum disorders (ASDs). The different diagnostic terms falling within the umbrella term of PDDs are as follows:

- Autistic disorder
- Asperger's disorder Pervasive developmental disorder not otherwise specified (PDD-NOS)
- Rett's disorder
- Childhood disintegrative disorder

AUTISTIC CHARACTERISTICS

An individual with autism may exhibit some of the following characteristics and these can range from mild to severe impairment.

- Social Interaction
  - Shows little interest and/or difficulty relating to people and the environment
  - Shows little or no eye contact
  - Prefers to be alone
  - Appears to live in own world
  - Does not seek comfort or affection
- Communication
  - Has unusual, delayed, or lack of spoken language (e.g., echolalia, use of gibberish)
  - Has difficulties with using and understanding language (e.g., expressing needs)
  - Misinterprets or misses nonverbal language (e.g., body language, gestures, facial expressions)
- Unusual Behaviors, Characteristics, and Interests
  - Unusual play with toys and other objects (e.g., spinning objects, obsessive attachment to toy/object or parts of a object)
  - Resistance to change (e.g., routine, environment)
  - Regulation of emotions (laughing, crying, distressed)

TABLE 1.1	DSM–IV–TR Diagnostic Criteria for Pervasive Developmental Disorders

Diagnostic Criteria for 299.00 Autistic Disorder

I. A total of six (or more) items from (1), (2), and (3), with at least two from (1), and one each from (2) and (3):

   A. Qualitative impairment in social interaction, as manifested by at least two of the following:

      1. Marked impairment in the use of multiple nonverbal behaviors such as eye-to-eye gaze, facial expression, body postures, and gestures to regulate social interaction

      2. Failure to develop peer relationships appropriate to developmental level

      3. A lack of spontaneous seeking to share enjoyment, interests, or achievements with other people (e.g., by a lack of showing, bringing, or pointing out objects of interest to other people)

      4. Lack of social or emotional reciprocity

II. Qualitative impairments in communication as manifested by at least one of the following:

   A. Delay in, or total lack of, the development of spoken language (not accompanied by an attempt to compensate through alternative modes of communication such as gesture or mime)

   B. In individuals with adequate speech, marked impairment in the ability to initiate or sustain a conversation with others

   C. Stereotyped and repetitive use of language or idiosyncratic language

   D. Lack of varied, spontaneous make-believe play or social imitative play appropriate to developmental level

III. Restricted repetitive and stereotyped patterns of behavior, interests, and activities, as manifested by at least one of the following:

   A. Encompassing preoccupation with one or more stereotyped and restricted patterns of interest that is abnormal either in intensity or in focus

   B. Apparently inflexible adherence to specific, nonfunctional routines or rituals

   C. Stereotyped and repetitive motor manners (e.g., hand or finger flapping or twisting, or complex whole-body movements)

   D. Persistent preoccupation with parts of objects

IV. Delays or abnormal functioning in at least one of the following areas, with onset prior to age 3 years: (1) social interaction, (2) language as used in social communication, or (3) symbolic or imaginative play

V. The disturbance is not better accounted for by Rett's disorder or childhood disintegrative disorder

Diagnostic Criteria for 299.80 Asperger's Disorder

I. Qualitative impairment in social interaction, as manifested by at least two of the following:

   A. Marked impairment in the use of multiple nonverbal behaviors such as eye-to eye gaze, facial expression, body postures, and gestures to regulate social interaction

   B. Failure to develop peer relationships appropriate to developmental level

   C. A lack of spontaneous seeking to share enjoyment, interests, or achievements with other people (e.g., by a lack of showing, bringing, or pointing out objects of interest to other people)

   D. Lack of social or emotional reciprocity

II. Restricted repetitive and stereotyped patterns of behavior, interests, and activities, as manifested by at least one of the following:

   A. Encompassing preoccupation with one or more stereotyped and restricted patterns of interest that is abnormal either in intensity or in focus

   B. Apparently inflexible adherence to specific, nonfunctional routines or rituals

   C. Stereotyped and repetitive motor mannerisms (e.g., hand or finger flapping or twisting, or complex whole-body movements)

   D. Persistent preoccupation with parts of objects

III. The disturbance causes clinically significant impairment in social, occupational, or other important areas of functioning

IV. There is no clinically significant general delay in language (e.g., single words used by age 2 years, communicative phrases used by age 3 years)

(continued)

TABLE 1.1	**DSM–IV–TR Diagnostic Criteria for Pervasive Developmental Disorders** *(continued)*

V. There is no clinically significant delay in cognitive development or in the development of age-appropriate self-help skills, adaptive behavior (other than in social interaction), and curiosity about the environment in childhood

VI. Criteria are not met for another specific pervasive developmental disorder or schizophrenia

Diagnostic Criteria for 299.80 Pervasive Developmental Disorder Not Otherwise Specified (Including Atypical Autism)

This category should be used when there is a severe and pervasive impairment in the development of reciprocal social interaction associated with impairment in either verbal or nonverbal communication skills or with the presence of stereotyped behavior, interests, and activities, but the criteria are not met for a specific pervasive developmental disorder, schizophrenia, schizotypal personality disorder, or avoidant personality disorder.

Diagnostic Criteria for 299.80 Rett's Disorder

I. All of the following:
   A. Apparently normal prenatal and perinatal development
   B. Apparently normal psychomotor development through the first 5 months after birth
   C. Normal head circumference at birth

II. Onset of all of the following after the period of normal development:
   A. Deceleration of head growth between ages 5 and 48 months
   B. Loss of previously acquired purposeful hand skills between ages 5 and 30 months with the subsequent development of stereotyped hand movements (e.g., hand-wringing or hand washing)
   C. Loss of social engagement early in the course (although often social interaction develops later)
   D. Appearance of poorly coordinated gait or trunk movements
   E. Severely impaired expressive and receptive language development with severe psychomotor retardation

Diagnostic Criteria for 299.10 Childhood Disintegrative Disorder

I. Apparently normal development for at least the first 2 years after birth as manifested by the presence of age-appropriate verbal and nonverbal communication, social relationships, play, and adaptive behavior

II. Clinically significant loss of previously acquired skills (before age 10 years) in at least two of the following areas:
   A. Expressive or receptive language
   B. Social skills or adaptive behavior
   C. Bowel or bladder control
   D. Play
   E. Motor skills

III. Abnormalities of functioning in at least two of the following areas:
   A. Qualitative impairment in social interaction (e.g., impairment in nonverbal behaviors, failure to develop peer relationships, lack of social or emotional reciprocity)
   B. Qualitative impairments in communication (e.g., delay or lack of spoken language, inability to initiate or sustain a conversation, stereotyped and repetitive use of language, lack of varied make-believe play)
   C. Restricted, repetitive, and stereotyped patterns of behavior, interest, and activities, including motor stereotypes and mannerisms

IV. The disturbance is not better accounted for by another specific pervasive developmental disorder or by schizophrenia

DSM–IV–TR, Diagnostic and Statistical Manual of Mental Disorders–Fourth Edition Text Revision.

- Behavioral issues (e.g., tantrums, aggressiveness, self-injurious)
- Sensory sensitivities (e.g., over or under pain sensitivity, loud and/or sudden noises, lights, food/fabric textures)
- Apparent oversensitivity or undersensitivity to pain
- Extreme high or low motoric activity level
- Lack of awareness of danger (e.g., runs into street, bolts in crowds)
- Stereotypic behaviors (e.g., rocking, spinning, finger/hand flapping)
- Limited and/or repetitive play skills
- Narrow range of interests

AUTISTIC SPECTRUM DISORDERS

Individuals with ASDs (also called PDDs) can exhibit associated characteristics and behaviors in degrees of severity and varying capabilities from mild to disabling. Some individuals may have slight delays or difficulties in one area, while having greater challenges in others. An example of this may be a child who makes eye contact but on an inconsistent basis or a child who has mild language difficulties but has difficulties with social interaction or has repetitive or obsessive behaviors. Children who are mildly affected may be diagnosed later than others, as well as children with more debilitating handicaps that may mask the characteristics associated with ASDs.

The remaining disorders under the umbrella term ASDs/PDDs are as follows.

ASPERGER'S DISORDER

Asperger's disorder was recognized in the *DSM–IV* in 1994, 50 years after Hans Asperger first wrote of this disorder (11). Characteristics of Asperger's disorder include the following:

- Less severe impairment in socialization and communication than in autism
- No clinically significant delays in
  - language,
  - cognitive development (average to superior intelligence),
  - self-help skills, or
  - adaptive behavior (other than in social interaction).
- Lack of social skills, such as social or emotional reciprocity; social awkwardness
- Restricted range of interests
- Difficulties understanding language subtleties such as satire or humor
- Speech patterns may be unusual (may speak in a monotone nature/lack inflection, may be too loud or high pitched

PERVASIVE DEVELOPMENTAL DISORDER (PDD)-NOS

The term PDD-NOS (sometimes referred to as atypical autism) is used when the diagnostic criteria are not fully met for a specific PDD, schizophrenia, schizotypal personality disorder, or avoidant personality disorder.

RETT'S DISORDER

Rett's disorder (also known as Rett's syndrome) is relatively rare, affecting almost exclusively women. Occurrence is noted to be 1 out of 10,000 to 15,000. Characteristics include the following:

- Initial development normal
- Onset between 6 and 18 months (may not be noticeable until 1–4 years of age)
- Progressive degeneration (begins 1–4 years of age) in mental, behavioral, social, and gross motor abilities

- Severe loss of communication
- Distinctive hand movements (wringing)

CHILDHOOD DISINTEGRATIVE DISORDER

Childhood disintegrative disorder is an extremely rare disorder. It is a clearly apparent regression in multiple areas of functioning:

- Initial development normal for a period of at least 2 years
- Average age of onset is between 3 and 4 years
- Onset can be gradual or sudden
- Progressive degeneration in all areas, such as the following:
  - Cognitive ability
  - Communication (expressive or receptive language)
  - Motor skills

TABLE 1.2	*Diagnostic and Statistical Manual of Mental Disorders* (*DSM*) Timeline on Autism

1. *DSM*

The original *DSM* was released in 1952. Autism was not included as a separate diagnostic condition, but characteristics now associated with autism spectrum disorders were included under the Schizophrenia, Childhood Type Disorder category.

2. *DSM–II*

The *DSM–II* was released in 1968, but autism continued not to be mentioned but is mentioned in the Schizophrenia, Childhood Type Disorder category, stating "this category is for cases in which schizophrenic symptoms appear before puberty … condition may be manifested by autistic, atypical and withdrawn behavior; failure to develop identity separate from the mother's; and general unevenness, gross immaturity and inadequacy in development."

3. *DSM–III*

Progress was seen when the *DSM–III* was released in 1980. The term "infantile autism" appeared as a diagnostic category and was no longer considered a psychiatric disorder but rather a developmental one. There were only six characteristics listed (e.g., onset before 30 months of age, language and developmental deficits); however, each of these symptoms was required to be present for diagnosis. Along with infantile autism was the category of Childhood Onset Pervasive Development Disorder. The *DSM–III–Revised* (*DSM–III–R*) was published in 1987. Pervasive developmental disorder became only two disorders in the revision, listing autistic disorder and pervasive developmental disorder not otherwise specified (PDD-NOS). Infantile autism was changed to autistic disorder. The diagnostic criteria for autism were more in depth, being defined by 16 criteria that were grouped into three areas of impairment (i.e., socialization, communication, and restricted range of interests and behaviors). The PDD-NOS term was broader and was used when individuals met only a few of the autism criteria. With the less restrictive criteria for a *DSM–III–R* diagnosis of autistic disorder, more children and adults were diagnosed with autism.

4. *DSM–IV/DSM–IV–TR*

DSM–IV was released in 1994 and the text revision (*DSM–IV–TR*) in 2000. The *DSM–IV* introduced the umbrella category of pervasive developmental disorders (PDDs). The *DSM–IV–TR* does not include any changes in this category. Along with autistic disorder, Asperger's disorder (also referred to as Asperger's syndrome or AS), Rett's disorder, childhood disintegrative disorder, and pervasive developmental disorder not otherwise specified (PDD-NOS) also came under the umbrella term of PDDs. Diagnostic criteria for Asperger's disorder were introduced with the *DSM–IV* edition.

5. *DSM–V*

The *DSM–V* is scheduled for publication in 2011.

- Social skills
- Bowel/bladder control
- Self-care
- Restricted, repetitive, stereotypic behaviors and interests

DIAGNOSIS

ASDs can often be reliably recognized by age 3. New research and comprehensive diagnostic tools are enabling specialists to detect the characteristics associated with the diagnosis of ASDs as early as 6 months to 1 year of age. Parents are often the first to notice their child's

- unusual behaviors;
- delay or failure to reach developmental milestones;
- unresponsiveness to people;
- intense and prolonged obsession with an object or part of an object; and/or
- regression of previously attained skills.

Although the diagnosis of ASDs in a young child certainly should be completed in a multidisciplinary and comprehensive manner, there is substantial evidence that early identification is paramount in order for a child to receive the specialized intervention for optimal results.

The intent behind the *DSM–IV–TR* is that the diagnostic criteria not be used as a checklist but, rather, as guidelines for diagnosing PDDs/ASDs, which are considered spectrum disorders, indicating that the associated characteristics and behaviors such as communication and social difficulties can occur on a continuum from mild to severe.

According to the definition set forth in the *DSM–IV* (10), PDDs are characterized by severe and pervasive impairment in several areas of development (see Table 1.2):

- Social interaction skills;
- Communication skills; or
- The presence of stereotyped behavior, interests, and activities.

REFERENCES

1. Autism PDD Support Network. History of autism. Retrieved May 29, 2009, from http://www.autism-pdd.net/autism-history.html
2. Developmental Behavioral Pediatrics. (2004). Autism. Retrieved June 5, 2009, from http://www.dbpeds.org/articles/detail.cfm?TextID=%2049
3. Hincha-Ownby M. (2008). History of autism in the DSM. Retrieved June 19, 2009, from http://autismaspergerssyndrome.suite101.com/article.cfm/history_of_autism_in_the_dsm
4. Kantrowitz B, Scelfo J. (2006). What happens when they grow up. *Newsweek.* Retrieved March 15, 2009, from http://www.newsweek.com/id/44634
5. Long W. (2007). The first clinical description of autism: Leo Kanner. Retrieved June 19, 2009, from http://www.drbilllong.com/Autism/Kanner.html
6. Williams R. (2000). Autism through ages baffles sciences. Retrieved May 19, 2009, from http://www.pediatricservices.com/prof/prof-26.htm
7. Autism Society of Washington. (2008). The history of autism. Retrieved May 29, 2009, from www.autismsocietyofwa.org
8. American Academy of Neurology Foundation. (2009). Autism. Retrieved June 5, 2009, from http://www.thebrainmatters.org/disorders/index.cfm?event=view&disorder_id=85
9. Centers for Disease Control and Prevention. Autism spectrum disorders. Retrieved November 3rd, 2010 from http://www.cdc.gov/ncbddd/autism/
10. American Psychiatric Association. *Diagnostic and Statistical Manual of Mental Disorders.* 4th ed., text revision. Washington, D.C.: American Psychiatric Association; 2000.
11. American Psychiatric Association. *Diagnostic and Statistical Manual of Mental Disorders.* 4th ed. Washington, D.C.: American Psychiatric Association; 1994.

Current Thoughts Regarding the Neurobiology of Autism

Autistic spectrum disorders (ASD) constitute a broad continuum of brain illnesses and range from exceptionally severe to very mild presentations. All these disorders share common clinical and behavioral features, but typically differ in severity and age of onset. Autism, the most severe of the disorders, begins in childhood and impairs thinking, feeling, language, and the ability to play and relate to others (1).

Diagnosis, training, and early intervention continue to be the key to the most successful outcomes that have been reported thus far. Landmark legislation, the Children's Health Act of 2000, mandated the National Institute of Mental Health (NIMH) to expand and coordinate research into autism causes and treatments. The Studies to Advance Autism Research and Treatment (STAART) is a network of several National Institutes of Health (NIH)–supported centers across the country. These centers conduct basic and clinical research, and include research in the fields of developmental neurobiology, genetics, clinical developmental psychology, and psychopharmacology. Although each center has a particular focus of research, information gathered from all centers may include research from postmortem brains, brain imaging, genetics, and animal studies.

NEUROANATOMIC RESEARCH

Clinical observations from the time of Kanner have yielded consistent findings that fail to translate into understanding of why the condition occurs. For instance, from Kanner's initial description of the disorder (1943), it has been commonly observed that the head circumferences of children with autism run larger than normal. Noninvasive brain imaging techniques offer enormous potential for understanding the complex mechanisms associated with ASD. Currently, research is directed at attempting not only to identify abnormalities, but also to better define normal growth curves of brain structures involved in the circuitry for language, thinking, and other functions. One such longitudinal study revealed a wave of neuronal overproduction in the frontal lobes prior to puberty in normal brains that had not been well appreciated before (2). By contrast, a wave of abnormal brain enlargement seen in MRI studies of young children with autism follows a back-to-front pattern similar to a wave of abnormal gray matter loss seen in childhood-onset schizophrenia, which suggests a process in which the timing and trajectory of various abnormalities parallel clinical outcome (2,3). Animal models continue to implicate key limbic structures, specifically the amygdala and hippocampus, as involved in the social and emotional abnormalities that are often impaired in individuals with ASD. Other animal research has implicated the development of milder autistic features when the medial temporal lobe was removed early in life (4). Processing itself is different in autistic minds, because there is a clear predilection for facts rather than fiction, as well as clear tendency to file information in separate rather than conceptually or semantically related folders (5). Further, the issue of emotions is complex, in that people with autism experience a wide range of emotions but it tends to be expressed in atypical ways with mouthing, hand flapping, and motor overflow (6).

Webb and Jones (7) have done careful studies tracking not only the clear increase of head circumference in the first 2 years of life, but that a surprising shrinkage of brain is ultimately found in those individuals with autistic behaviors by end of the adult years. At least some theories exist which suggest that exuberance of neuronal dendritic branching is not kept adequately in check as in normally developing children, leading to an excessive amount of dendritic arborization with inadequate pruning, the quintessential "overgrown garden" metaphor that is sometimes used to describe the morphologic changes in the brains of these children in the first 2 years of life. Using computerized sections of sections of cortex, investigators have found that the vertical columns of the six histologically distinct layers seen in children with autism are often smaller, with less dense, but spikier, neurons than in controls (5). One of the more exciting areas of research involves the discovery of locally inflamed microglia in the first 2 years of life of children with autism (8). Because these regions resemble the brains of adult patients with Alzheimer's disease, it is hoped that drug interaction at the level of reducing such inflammation might have the potential for preventing long-term damage of the actively deteriorating brain in autism.

Brains of people with autism also have disordered myelin. The work of Minshew (9) has shown that the corpus callosum is often much smaller than in controls. Because myelin is the part of the neuron essential for the rapid transmission of impulses, it is theorized that underdevelopment of the corpus callosum and other large myelin bundles in the central nervous system (CNS) may contribute to the complex autistic patterns of behavior. Certainly, the brain stem is frequently the target of many investigators. Many investigators have found decreased volume of tissue in the deep cerebellar nuclei, specifically the emboliform, the fastigial, the globose, and the dentate, as well as the nuclei of the brain stem proper, such as the superior and inferior olive, locus coeruleus, arcuate nuclei, and the facial nucleus itself (10–12).

GENETIC INVESTIGATIONS

The genetics of autism is complex. Up to 100 or more genetic variations of autism have been described, with as many as four or more alleles implicated on each chromosome (13). Recently, four previously undetected chromosomal sites strongly linked to autism have been discovered by investigators at Columbia University and the University of Oxford, which added regions on chromosomes 2, 6, 8, and 17 to the growing list of areas most suspicious for autism-predisposing genes. The same research added additional evidence to known areas of chromosomes 7, 16, and 19 (14). The genetic investigation of autism is hampered considerably not only by the wide phenotypical presentation of autism, but also by the complexity of knowing what tissue to study and at what age of life. Any genetic mutation in the context of autism can be considered to be twofold in its influence: the genetic mutation itself and the cascade effect it generates throughout the rest of the CNS. Although the technique of finding a single gene defect can be measured using standard techniques, such as Northern blotting or reverse transcription with polymerase chain reaction, tracking the effects of a genetic mutation through other systems is far more complex. The use of DNA (deoxyribonucleic acid) microarray technology has been applied to many neurologic conditions, including autism, and has been instrumental in identifying the influence of those genetic problems encountered in fragile X and Rett's syndrome—two conditions that both express the phenotypical traits of autism (15). The condition of autism is itself so heterogeneous as to present a real challenge to know which "flavor" of autism is most representational of the whole. Indeed, whole-genome linkage scans suggest that the prototypic autistic disorder is likely to be caused by changes in many genes, across several chromosomes (16).

Apart from the autosomal chromosomes, the X chromosome is also strongly associated with autism. Fragile X is the most common inherited cause of mental retardation, and frequently presents not only with mental retardation but also with classic features of the autistic phenotype (17). The absence of the paternal X chromosome has been implicated rather than that of the Y chromosome, for several reasons, among which is that girls with only an X, O karyotype, or Turner's syndrome, may have mild-to-moderate intellectual impairment but rarely present with autistic features (18).

The abnormal migration of neural crest cells has been implicated in many and varied diseases, and autism is no exception. Neural crest migrational defects are responsible for neurocutaneous diseases, including neurofibromatosis and tuberous sclerosis (TS)—the latter far more commonly associated with autism than the former. TS is a tumor-suppressor gene syndrome with an incidence of 1 in 10,000. TS presents with a wide range of both malignant and benign tumors, and depending on the survey, from one-third to two-thirds of all patients with TS present with autism. Although the genes that most commonly cause TS, hamartin (9q34) and tuberin (16p13), are well known, it is less clear what specifically about the genes themselves produce the autistic behavioral phenotype commonly seen in TS (18). Theories include the following: first, a secondary effect from the typical and devastating seizures that are often seen in children with TS, specifically infantile spasms; second, a susceptibility gene for autism that becomes activated in the presence of a TS gene; and third, the direct effect of the TS gene early in neurogenesis may create the similar phenotype of autism, apart from any stimulation of autism activation genes (19).

SUBCELLULAR AND NEUROTRANSMITTER INVESTIGATIONS

Neurotransmitters have been studied extensively in autism. Catecholamines especially have been a rich source of interest for researchers because of the involvement in behavior disturbances seen in autism, such as "motor control, reward, cognition, stereopathies, obsessional relations with objects, hyperactivity, attention," and sleep alterations (19). Investigations have included looking not only at the synthesis of the transmitters, but also at the receptor sites and malformations involved. Serotonin (5-hydroxytryptamine or 5-HT) has been implicated in a wide range of disorders, which included derangements of mood, social phobias, and obsessive–compulsive disorders (20).

With the current emphasis on the role of cerebellar circuitry, attention is focused on the GABAergic system, because gamma-aminobutyric acid (GABA) is the most common neurotransmitter in that system. GABA is critical to mediating the interneurons in the hippocampus and limbic system and their ultimate connections in a loop back to the Purkinje cells of the cerebellum. Candidate genes for the structure of GABA, specifically GABRβ3, have been found to be strongly associated with the 15q11-13 region of the genetic map, and may ultimately yield a clue about the role of GABA-mediated pathology in autism (21).

Cholinergic dysfunction has been well described in autism as well, and includes the fact that although there is no difference in choline acetyltransferase (ChAT) or acetylcholinesterase activity in the cerebral cortex or basal forebrain in patients with autism, there are profound differences seen at the level in the cerebellum, specifically in the sheer numbers of the $\alpha4\beta2$-subtype nicotinic receptors that are deficient in number and quality, with a nearly threefold increase in other types, specifically the $\alpha7$ nicotinic subtype (22).

Reelin is a large protein produced from a site on chromosome 7 that has been clearly found to be implicated in several psychiatric conditions, including bipolar and schizophrenia. The discovery of this rather large protein in 1995 generated a great deal of excitement because of how it directly affects several neurotransmitter systems. Subsequently, some sets of monozygotic twins with autism have also been found to have mutated forms of the reelin protein (23). The implication that significant learning disabilities as well as syndromes, among them autism, could be pinpointed to a single neurotransmitter-altering protein is enormous. Larger replications of these early studies will be critical to further elucidate the role of the reelin protein in psychiatric disorders.

THE IMMUNE SYSTEM AND AUTISM

Finally, the immune system in autism continues to be a hotly debated area of research. As alluded to earlier, exciting evidence exists that correlates the heightened activity of microglial cells in the cortex in the first 2 years of life in children with autism, much like one would see in older adults with Alzheimer's disease, giving rise to the thought that autism is also a neurodegenerative disease that occurs early in life (7). Microglia are activated when there is debris to be cleared from the destruction of CNS cells. Although a certain level of microglial activity is normal in children, the degree to which it has been seen in children with autism suggests the activation of a major histocompatibility complex that is potentially responsive to steroids and other anti-inflammatory agents. Although there are anecdotal reports of improvements, no placebo-controlled trials of these therapies have been reported (24).

REFERENCES

1. National Institute of Health/Interagency Coordination Committee Research Matrix (NIH/IACC). (2006). Retrieved National Institute of Mental Health. (2010). Autism Spectrum Disorders (Pervasive Developmental Disorders). Retrieved November 3rd, 2010 from http://www.nimh.nih.gov/health/topics/autism-spectrum-disorders-pervasive-developmental-disorders/index.shtml

2. Giedd JN, Blumenthal J, Jeffries NO, et al. Brain development during childhood and adolescence: a longitudinal MRI study. *Nat Neurosci*. 1999;2:861–863.

3. Courchesne E, Carper R, Akshoomoff N. Evidence of brain overgrowth in the first year of life in autism. *J Am Med Assoc*. 2003;290:337–344.

4. Bachevalier J, Malkova, L, Mishkin M. Effects of selective neonatal temporal lobe lesions on socioemotional behavior in infant rhesus monkeys. *Behav Neurosci*. 2001;115:545–559.

5. Bauman ML, Kemper TL. *The Neurobiology of Autism*. 2nd ed. Baltimore: Johns Hopkins University Press; 2005.

6. Bryson SE, Wainwright-Sharp A, Smith IM. Autism: a spatial neglect syndrome? In: Enns J, ed. *The Development of Attention: Research and Theory*. Amsterdam: Elsevier; 1990:405–427.

7. Webb SJ, Jones EJH. Early identification of autism: early characteristics, onset of symptoms, and diagnostic stability. *Infant Young Child*. 2009;22:100–118.

8. Courchesne E. The cerebellum in autism. *North Texas Summit on Autism*. Dallas, TX: University of Texas Southwestern School of Medicine, Department of Psychiatry; November 11, 2006.

9. Minshew NJ. Understanding Asperger syndrome and high functioning autism. *Int J Res Pract*. 2003;7:331–333.

10. Bauman ML, Kemper TL. Neuroanatomic observations in autism. In: Bauman ML, Kemper TL, eds. *The Neurobiology of Autism*. Baltimore: Johns Hopkins University Press; 1994:119–145.

11. Bailey A, Luthert P, Dean A. A clinicopathological study of autism. *Brain*. 1998;121:889–905.

12. Rodier P, Bryson S, Welch J. Minor physical anomalies and physical measurements in autism: data from Nova Scotia. *Teratology*. 1997;9:319–325.

13. Cook E. The genetics of autism. *North Texas Summit on Autism*. Dallas, TX: University of Texas Southwestern School of Medicine, Department of Psychiatry; November 11, 2006.

14. International Molecular Genetic Study of Autism Consortium. A genomewide screen for autism: strong evidence for linkage to chromosomes 2q, 7q and 16p. *Am J Hum Genet*. 2001;69:570–581.

15. Brasma A, Vilo J. Gene expression data analysis. *FEBS Lett*. 2000;480:17–24.

16. Lamb J, Moore J, Eschoo M. Autism: recent molecular genetic advances. *Hum Mol Genet*. 2001;9:861–868.

17. Hagerman R, Jackson A, Levitas A. An analysis of autism in fifty males with the fragile X syndrome. *Am J Med Genet*. 1986;23:359–374.

18. Smalley S. Autism and tuberous sclerosis, *J Autism Dev Disord*. 2008;28:407–414.

19. Holden J, Liu X. The role of dopamine and norepinephrine in autism; from behavior and pharmacotherapy to genetics. In: Bauman ML, Kemper TL, eds. *The Neurobiology of Autism*. Baltimore, MD: Johns Hopkins Press; 2005:276–299.

20. Anderson G. Monoamines in autism: an update of neurochemical research on pervasive developmental disorder. *Med Biol*. 1987;65:67–74.

21. Blatt GJ, Fitzgerald CM, Guptill JT, Brooker AB, Kemper TL, Bauman ML. Density and distribution of hippocampal neurotransmitter receptors in autism: an autoradiographic study. *J Autism Dev Disord*. 2001;31I:537–543.

22. Perry EK, Lee ML, Martin-Ruiz CM, et al. Cholinergic activities in autism: abnormalities in the cerebral cortex and basal forebrain, *Am J Psychiatry*. 2001;158:1058–1066.

23. Fatemi S, Stary J, Egan E. Defective Reelin production as a vulnerability factor in genesis of autism. *Cell Mol Neurobiol*. 2002;22:139–152.

24. Zimmerman A. Commentary: immunological treatments for autism: in search of reasons for promising approaches. *J Autism Dev Disord*. 2000;30:481–484.

3 Changing Demographics of Autism in the United States

There is vigorous and continued discussion on whether the current epidemic of individuals with a diagnosis under the autistic spectrum actually represents a true increase in the prevalence of autism (1). The current prevalence of 1 per 110 children who have an autistic spectrum disorder (ASD) most likely represents both an increase in numbers of cases as well as changes in criteria over the last 15 years to include milder cases as well represents an increase, although it is unclear why. The increase can be partly attributed to changes in the criteria used to diagnose autism along with increased recognition of the disorder by professionals and the public may all be contributing to the increased prevalence as currently reported. Regardless, the Centers for Disease Control and Prevention (CDC) confirms that children are being diagnosed with ASD more than any time before in this country.

Currently, using the broader definitions found in the Diagnostic and Statistical Manual of Mental Disorders—Fourth Edition (DSM–IV), the CDC estimates that between 2 and 6 children per 1,000, or approximately ranging from 1 in 500 to 1 in 112 children, have a diagnosis under the ASD spectrum. This is indeed alarming, given that although lower than rates for childhood mental retardation at approximately 10 per 1,000 children, an ASD diagnosis occurs more frequently than cerebral palsy at 2.8 per 1,000 children, hearing loss at 1.1 per 1,000 children, and visual impairment at 0.9 per 1,000 children (2). The male-to-female ratio varies from 1.33:1 to 16.0:1, with a mean of 4.4:1. The male excess is more pronounced when autism is not associated with mental retardation, and in such cases, approached 6:1 (3). At least some studies suggest that the high prevalence of males to females is an X-linked disorder, although the data supporting this are still quite sketchy (4). The overall proportion of cases of autism that can be directly linked to medical causes is actually quite low, approximately 6%. The most commonly associated medical disorders with autism include the neurocutaneous disorders such as tuberous sclerosis and neurofibromatosis, fragile X syndrome, Tourette's syndrome, phenylketonuria, congenital rubella, and Down's syndrome (3).

REFERENCES

1. Autism and Developmental Disabilities Monitoring Network Surveillance Year 2002 Principal Investigators; Centers for Disease Control and Prevention. Prevalence of autism spectrum disorders: autism and developmental disabilities. Monitoring network, 14 sites, United States, 2002. *Mor Mortal Wkly Rep CDC Surveill Summ*. 2007;56:12–28.
2. Yeargin-Allsopp M, Rice C, Karapurka T, Doernberg N, Boyle C, Murphy C. Prevalence of autism in a U.S. Metropolitan area. *J Am Med Assoc*. 2003;289:49–55.
3. Fombonne E. The epidemiology of pervasive developmental disorders. In: Baum ML, Kemper TL, eds. *The Neurobiology of Autism*. Baltimore, MD: Johns Hopkins Press; 2005:5–19.
4. Hagerman R, Jackson A, Levitas A. An analysis of autism in fifty males with the fragile X syndrome. *Am J Med Genet*. 1986;23:359–374.

Incorporating People with Autism within the Primary Care Practice

4

Primary care physicians (PCPs) encounter the broadest possible scope of patients. In the context of the sweeping epidemic of autistic spectrum disorders (ASD), it is inevitable that anyone in the primary care services, can expect ultimately take care of an individual with an ASD. What is critically important is for the PCP to understand how autism colors the physical and social health of the individual as well.

PCPs may wonder how to most appropriately incorporate these individuals into a busy primary care office. It is the genuine hope of these authors that this text will provide ways to adopt simple screening and clinical techniques that can streamline a clinician's need to identify, medically support, and provide long-term care for individuals with autism.

Rapid screening for individuals can be obtained at the time of new patient assessment and for those established patients who may have missed initial screening. If the diagnosis of an ASD is suspected but not confirmed, assessments are available free until age 22 through the public school system, state and national organizations, or in specialized clinical settings (1). However, PCPs have access to a wide range of psychometric instruments, primarily questionnaires, which can guide the diagnosis, although they are not necessarily confirmatory (2–5). Such instruments are widely available commercially and easily administered in the PCP setting (6–25). The majority of adults would be expected to have been diagnosed with ASD during their academic years. These individuals will be assisted through transition programs into adult services through public school special education mandates, often including local/state/federal agencies. Many of the state and government programs require that a person has a mental or physical impairment that substantially hinders skills such as self-care, independent living, economic self-sufficiency, and communication. Private insurance may pay for part or all of private evaluations, but because of the expense, this should be investigated prior to committing to assessments that the patient may not be able to afford.

Once diagnosed, one of the most labor-intensive steps is taking time to visit at length and in an unhurried fashion which symptoms are most distressing to the patient and/or family. Many high-functioning individuals with Asperger's syndrome may successfully marry and hold highly technical jobs, but still struggle with intrusive obsessive tendencies that may be sensitive to an anxiolytic. Conversely, a nonverbal, highly aggressive, chronically disruptive 5-year-old may need a neuroleptic at low doses to provide significant relief for all involved. Having patients wait months to years for a subspecialist to become available should be reserved for patients who present diagnostic and therapeutic challenges not relieved by a few straightforward clinical approaches.

Subsequently, the best reasons for developing a primary care practice that actively recruits and cares for individuals with ASD diagnoses include the following:

- Providing immediate relief with often dramatic improvement in quality of life using primary care–level therapeutics and medication.
- Enriching the practitioner's professional experience by knowing and caring for a segment of the population that is often neglected, but consists often of delightfully interesting and truly unique individuals.
- Anticipating and preparing for the 1 in 112 individuals who presents with an ASD in a careful and systematic way alleviates the inevitable stress a primary care practice office might otherwise experience.

In conclusion, the sheer prevalence of individuals with ASD predicts that most primary care practitioners will encounter significant numbers of patients with autism or Asperger's syndrome. With incorporation of simple screening techniques and adoption of a few strategies for clinical management, pediatricians, family practitioners, obstetricians, and internists can make the care of individuals with autism one of the most challenging, interesting, and gratifying aspect of their practice.

REFERENCES

1. U.S. Department of Education. Building the legacy: IDEA 2004. Retrieved November 3rd, 2010 from http://idea.ed.gov/explore/home
2. American Academy of Pediatrics, Council on Children With Disabilities, Section on Developmental and Behavioral Pediatrics, Bright Futures Steering Committee, Medical Home Initiatives for Children With Special Needs Project Advisory Committee. Identifying infants and young children with developmental disorders in the medical home: an algorithm for developmental surveillance and screening. *Pediatrics*. 2006;118:405–420. [Published correction appears in *Pediatrics*. 2006;119:1808–1809.]
3. Sand N, Silverstein M, Glascoe FP, Gupta VB, Tonniges TP, O'Connor KG. Pediatricians' reported practices regarding developmental screening: do guidelines work? Do they help? *Pediatrics*. 2005;116: 174–179.
4. Sices L, Feudtner C, McLaughlin J, Drotar D, Williams M. How do primary care physicians identify young children with developmental delays? A national survey. *J Dev Behav Pediatr*. 2003;24:409–417.
5. Gupta VB, Hyman SL, Johnson CP, et al. Identifying children with autism early. *Pediatrics*. 2007;119: 152–153. [Published correction appears in *Pediatrics*. 2007;119:867.]
6. Wetherby AM, Prizant BM. *Communication and Symbolic Behavior Scales Developmental Profile (CSBS DP): First Normed Edition*. Baltimore, MD: Paul H Brookes; 2002.
7. Dietz C, Swinkels S, van Daalen E, van Engeland H, Buitelaar JK. Screening for autistic spectrum disorder in children aged 14–15 months. II: population screening with the Early Screening of Autistic Traits Questionnaire (ESAT)—design and general findings. *J Autism Dev Disord*. 2006;36:713–722.
8. Swinkels SH, Dietz C, van Daalen E, Kerkhof IH, van Engeland H, Buitelaar JK. Screening for autistic spectrum disorder in children aged 14 to 15 months. I: the development of the Early Screening of Autistic Traits Questionnaire (ESAT). *J Autism Dev Disord*. 2006;36:723–732.
9. Coonrod EE, Stone WL. Screening for autism in young children. In: Volkmar FR, Paul R, Klin A, Cohen D, eds. *Handbook of Autism and Pervasive Developmental Disorders*. 3rd ed. Vol 2. Hoboken, NJ: John Wiley & Sons; 2005:707–729.
10. Lord C, Corsello C. Diagnostic instruments in autistic spectrum disorders. In: Volkmar FR, Paul R, Klin A, Cohen D, eds. *Handbook of Autism and Pervasive Developmental Disorders*. 3rd ed. Vol II. Hoboken, NJ: John Wiley & Sons; 2005:730–771.
11. Camp BW. What the clinician really wants to know: questioning the clinical usefulness of sensitivity and specificity in studies of screening tests. *J Dev Behav Pediatr*. 2006;27:226–230.
12. Baron-Cohen S, Allen J, Gillberg C. Can autism be detected at 18 months? The needle, the haystack, and the CHAT. *Br J Psychiatry*. 1992;161:839–843.
13. Robins D, Fein D, Barton M, Green JA. The Modified-Checklist for Autism in Toddlers (M-CHAT): an initial investigation in the early detection of autism and pervasive developmental disorders. *J Autism Dev Disord*. 2001;31:131–144.
14. Siegel B. *The Pervasive Developmental Disorders Screening Test II (PDDST-II)*. San Antonio, TX: Harcourt Assessment; 2004.
15. Campbell JM. Diagnostic assessment of Asperger's disorder: a review of five third-party rating scales. *J Autism Dev Disord*. 2005;35:25–35.
16. Williams J, Scott F, Stott C, et al. The CAST (Childhood Asperger Syndrome Test): test accuracy. *Autism*. 2005;9:45–68.
17. Schopler E, Reichler RJ, Rochen Renner B. *The Childhood Autism Rating Scale (CARS)*. Los Angeles, CA: Western Psychological Services; 1988.
18. Sevin JA, Matson JL, Coe DA, Fee VE, Sevin BM. A comparison and evaluation of three commonly used autism scales. *J Autism Dev Disord*. 1991;21:417–432.
19. Gilliam JE. *Gilliam Asperger's Disorder Scale (GADS)*. Austin, TX: Pro-Ed; 2001.
20. Gilliam JE. *Gilliam Autism Rating Scale 2nd Edition (GARS-2)*. Austin, TX: Pro-Ed; 2006.

21. Krug DA, Arick JR. *Krug Asperger's Disorder Index (KADI)*. Austin, TX: Pro-Ed; 2003.

22. Stone WL, Coonrod EE, Ousley OY. Brief report: Screening Tool for Autism in Two-Year-Olds (STAT): development and preliminary data. *J Autism Dev Disord.* 2000;30:607–612.

23. Stone WL, Coonrod EE, Turner LM, Pozdol SL. Psychometric properties of the STAT for early autism screening. *J Autism Dev Disord.* 2004;34:691–701.

24. Berument SK, Rutter M, Lord C, Pickles A, Bailey A. Autism screening questionnaire: diagnostic validity. *Br J Psychiatry.* 1999;175:444–451.

25. Rutter M, Bailey A, Lord C, et al. *The Social Communication Questionnaire (SCQ) Manual.* Los Angeles, CA: Western Psychological Services; 2003.

Section Two:

Symptom-Based Assessment

Algorithm for the Evaluation and Management of Individuals with Autistic Spectrum Disorders

5

TABLE 5.1	Flowchart for Evaluation and Management of Autistic Spectrum Disorders (ASDs) Based on Presenting Symptoms

I. *For all referrals of suspected ASDs*
  A. *Before examination*
    1. *Parents complete age-appropriate development screen on arrival to office*
    2. *May include a statement for parents to specifically state what they wish to accomplish for today's visit as regards behavior, academics, or developmental concerns*
  B. *History*
    1. *Perform Denver developmental screen II*
    2. *Review of any reported delay: verify slow (delayed) vs. loss of previously achieved skills (regression)*
    3. *Validate if newborn screening has been performed*
    4. *Perform careful family history, including risk for consanguinity or early postnatal deaths*
    5. *Perform careful perinatal history, with particular attention to gestation, birth weight, and any perinatal issues*
    6. *Obtain release for all school records, including any psychometric or standardized tests*
    7. *Review social history for degrees of opportunity the child has to socialize with peers*
  C. *Physical*
    1. *Observation of child with family and at play during history gathering*
    2. *Height, weight, and head circumference plotted and checked*
    3. *General examination with particular attention to possible dysmorphology; shape of spine, shape/size of head, and skin lesions*
    4. *Eye contact, which needs to be specifically described as appropriate, fleeting, or none*
    5. *Mental status examination, with particular attention to speech patterns, level of maturity relative to age, capacity to engage with the examiner, and capacity to be redirected as needed*
    6. *Neurologic examination with specific attention to eye examination, facial symmetry, quality of voice, dysmorphic features, optic discs if possible, visual fields; strength, tone, general sensory examination, gait, and coordination*
II. *Delay in children with autistic traits*
  A. *Speech delay*
    1. *Speech assessment (may need to include specific request for expressive, receptive, pragmatic, and/or syntactic speech delay)*
    2. *Hearing assessment (may require a bilateral auditory evoked response)*
      a. *If delayed, consider magnetic resonance imaging (MRI)*
      b. *Lead levels*
    3. *Referral to assistive technology as indicated*
    4. *Consider referral for social skills coaching as indicated to facilitate pragmatic speech*
  B. *Social*
    1. *Psychometric testing*
      a. *Consider Vineland Adaptive Behavior Scales, Second Edition (VABS-II), or the Adaptive Behavior Assessment System, Second Edition (ABAS-II); may need additional psychometric measures for cognitive assessment*
      b. *May need play therapy as support for other speech or occupational therapy (OT)*
      c. *Mild-to-severe social impairment may be seen in individuals with Asperger's syndrome, but relatively sophisticated speech may mask symptoms initially*

TABLE 5.1	Flowchart for Evaluation and Management of Autistic Spectrum Disorders (ASDs) Based on Presenting Symptoms *(continued)*

    2. *Speech assessment: request specifically for receptive and pragmatic speech*
    3. *OT for sensory integration, for the child who seems particularly oblivious to his environment*
  C. *Motor*
    1. *OT assessment: can provide very specific snapshot of skills relative to age, with specific goal-driven therapy*
    2. *Physical therapy assessment*
    3. *Serologies: Creatine Kinase (CK), especially prior to sedation for any investigation such as MRI*
  D. *Cognitive*
    1. *Psychometric testing*
      a. *Have family request meeting with school officials to discuss results*
      b. *Family should aim for maintaining cordial relationships with school, but attempt to have thorough and explicit remedies implemented*
      c. *Advise family to keep copies of all school meetings and test results*
    2. *Serologies: Fragile X genetic screen, consider either genetic testing or referral; further metabolic assessment as driven by findings on physical examination*
    3. *Imaging: consider imaging if neurologic evaluation suggests focal findings in addition to cognitive delay, including but not limited to concerns of head size, shape, or dysmorphologies*
III. *Odd behaviors in children with autistic traits (see Chapter 7)*
  A. *Sensory defensiveness/neediness*
    1. *Refer to OT for assessment*
    2. *Consider speech therapy if sensory issues revolve around feeding or oral motor problems*
      a. *No or insufficient improvement; consider either an <u>selective serotonin reuptake inhibitor</u> (SSRI) or an antipsychotic for exceptional problems*
      b. *Social awkwardness*
        1. *Refer to behavioral modification; consider cognitive therapy and/or virtual reality therapy for individuals with verbal, high-functioning, or Asperger's syndrome*
        2. *No or insufficient improvement; consider anxiolytic for exceptional problems*
  B. *Obsession and ritual*
    1. *Provide stable and predictable environment and routine*
    2. *Consider use of OT to coach self-soothing techniques, often in conjunction with behavioral therapy*
    3. *No or insufficient improvement; consider either an SSRI or an antipsychotic for exceptional problems*
  C. *Stereotypical behavior*
    1. *Provide stable and predictable environment and routine*
    2. *Consider use of OT to assist with redirection and refocusing if stereotypies are self-abusing or interfering with daily functioning*
    3. *No or insufficient improvement; consider either an SSRI or an antipsychotic for exceptional problems*
  D. *Self-abusing behavior*
    1. *Provide stable and predictable environment and routine*
    2. *Consider what provocations are particularly troublesome, and attempt to remove or change if possible*
    3. *Consider physical therapy consult for physical supports, such as helmets, arm splints, etc., to minimize harm*
    4. *Consider OT to find substitute items for self-soothing*
    5. *No or insufficient improvement; consider either an SSRI or an antipsychotic for exceptional problems*

TABLE 5.1	**Flowchart for Evaluation and Management of Autistic Spectrum Disorders (ASDs) Based on Presenting Symptoms** *(continued)*

IV. *Regression in children with autistic traits (see Chapter 8)*
   A. *Previously developmentally appropriate child now regressing with autistic features*
      1. *Neurophysiology*
         a. *All children with regression*
            1. *Routine electroencephalogram (EEG)*
               i. *Abnormal: refer to pediatric neurology for management*
               ii. *Normal: consider overnight or extended EEG tracing*
            2. *Overnight EEG*
               i. *Abnormal: refer to pediatric neurology*
               ii. *Normal: monitor clinically*
         b. *Hearing screen*
         c. *Vision screen*
   B. *Both cognitive and motor decline with elevated serum creatine kinase*
         1. *Nerve conduction/Motor conduction studies*
         2. *Referral to pediatric neuromuscular specialist*
         3. *Referral to genetics*
            i. *Imaging: MRI without contrast of head*
         a. *Normocephalic*
            1. *Abnormal: consider referral to pediatric neurology, genetics*
            2. *Normal: repeat only if clinical examination changes*
         b. *Macrocephalic*
            1. *Hydrocephalus: consider referral to pediatric neurosurgery*
            2. *Normal or atrophic: Alexander; Canavan*
      1. *Serologies*
         a. *Isolated decline of cognitive function*
            1. *Urine organic acids: galactosemia, Sanfillipo, Maple syrup urine*
               i. *Disease; homocysteinuria*
            2. *Serum amino acid: Histidinemia; homocysteinemia*
            3. *Serum chemistries: creatine kinase; liver function; complete blood count (CBC) with differential, lactate, pyruvate, carnitine*
            4. *Genetic screens: fragile X; chromosome analysis; DNA microarray*
         b. *Coarse facial features*
            1. *Thyroid function*
               i. *Hypothyroidism: refer to pediatric endocrinology*
               ii. *Euthyroid: Hurler phenotype: evaluate for*
      2. *Mucopolysaccharidoses*
         c. *Motor decline:*
            1. *Creatine kinase: if elevated, refer to pediatric neurology*
          d. *Skin changes*
            1. *Genetic evaluation as indicated for neurofibromatosis, tuberous sclerosis, or other neurocutaneous disorders*
         e. *HIV risk*
            1. *HIV testing*
            2. *Consider referral to pediatric infectious disease for more extensive testing*
V. *Problems related to eating and elimination in children with autistic traits (see Chapter 9)*
   A. *Problems with eating, or with eating a limited choice of foods*
      1. *Referral to speech therapy for swallowing study and/or therapeutic approach to oral motor weakness and/or sensory aversion*
      2. *Referral to nutritional consult for tracking caloric intake if weight loss is progressive*
      3. *Referral to behavior therapy for behavior modification to broaden exceptionally limiting diet*

(continued)

TABLE 5.1	Flowchart for Evaluation and Management of Autistic Spectrum Disorders (ASDs) Based on Presenting Symptoms *(continued)*

B. *Problems with sleeping*
  1. *Sleep calendar for at least 1 week and ideally 1 month*
  2. *Ensure good sleep hygiene: consistent bedtime, no televisions or electronic screens in bedroom, child has his own bed*
  3. *For seriously disturbed sleep in spite of good environmental measures, request sleep study; consider also a routine EEG*
  4. *For obstructive sleep issues, referral to ENT*
  5. *For nonobstructive sleep issues, consider the use of small dose of α-agonist, such as clonidine at bedtime to reduce sleep-onset latency*
  6. *For persistence in sleep disorders, consider referral either to pediatric pulmonology, neurology, or sleep specialist*
C. *Problems with elimination*
  1. *Toilet training*
    a. *Delay in toilet training: consider use of behavior management*
    b. *If toilet training is associated with phobias, consider the use of medication to reduce anxiety*
  2. *Inappropriate interest or play with toilet*
    a. *Consider use of behavior management specific to cognitive level*
    b. *Consider use of atypical neuroleptic and/or SSRI to reduce compulsivity*
VI. *ASD and epilepsy (see Chapter 10)*
  A. *Regression or delay of social, motor, language skills*
    1. *Routine EEG: ideally with both sleep and waking tracings*
      a. *If normal EEG, but with no evidence of typical events captured during the tracing, request extended EEG*
        1. *Normal extended EEG*
          i. *Pursue serologic and radiographic evaluation as indicated for regression of milestones*
          ii. *Consider repeating EEG if symptoms persist and are not correlated with existing EEGs*
        2. *Abnormal extended EEG*
          i. *Refer to pediatric neurology*
          ii. *Obtain head imaging, preferably MRI*
          iii. *Genetic evaluation*
          iv. *If anticonvulsants are required, should anticipate a team approach with the pediatric neurologist long term to assist with seizure choice, dosing, and long-term management*
      b. *Abnormal routine EEG*
        1. *Refer to pediatric neurology*
        2. *Obtain head imaging, ideally an MRI*
        3. *Genetic evaluation*
        4. *If anticonvulsants are required, should anticipate a team approach with the pediatric neurologist long term to assist with seizure choice, dosing, and long-term management*
VII. *Psychiatric problems in children with autistic traits (see Chapter 11)*
  A. *Aggression*
    1. *Determine if threat to self or others; if so, refer to Emergency Department (ED)*
    2. *If not, consider the use of appropriate medication, such as an atypical neuroleptic or anticonvulsant*
  B. *Anxiety*
    1. *Determine if threat to self or others; if so, refer to Emergency Department (ED)*
    2. *If not, consider the use of appropriate medication such as an atypical neuroleptic or SSRI*

TABLE 5.1	**Flowchart for Evaluation and Management of Autistic Spectrum Disorders (ASDs) Based on Presenting Symptoms** *(continued)*

    C. *Mood disorders*
        1. *Determine if threat to self or others; if so, refer to ED*
        2. *If not, consider the use of a mood stabilizer, such as an atypical neuroleptic or SSRI*
    D. *Psychoses*
        1. *Refer to psychiatric ED*
        2. *Anticipate the need for psychiatrist for long-term care*
        3. *Anticipate the need for psychiatrist for long-term care*
VIII. *Genetic and environmental syndromes associated with autistic traits (see Chapter 12)*
    A. *Fragile X*
        1. *Assess for FMR1 gene in all children with autism plus cognitive deficiency*
        2. *FMR1 carrier state (permutation) in females may be as symptomatic as full expression in males*
        3. *If an index case is found, genetic counseling must include the extended family*
    B. *Neurocutaneous disorders*
        1. *Tuberous sclerosis (TS)*
            a. *Two gene products, hamartin and tuberin, can produce the clinical picture*
            b. *Seizures may present before autistic features*
            c. *Although TS is an autosomal-dominant condition, most cases are spontaneous mutations. Nevertheless, genetic counseling is warranted if a TS index case is found*
        2. *Neurofibromatosis type 1 (NF1)*
            a. *Although less commonly associated with ASD than with Learning Disability (LD), NF1 nevertheless is linked*
            b. *NF1 is autosomal dominant, and if an index case is found, genetic counseling is needed*
    C. *Phenylketonuria*
        1. *Usually identified in newborn screening*
        2. *In the context of microcephaly, delay, musty order, and possibility of a missed newborn screen, this should be considered*
    D. *Angelman syndrome (AS)*
        1. *Flourescent In-Situ Hybridization (FISH) for 15q deletion syndrome should be requested in cognitively delayed, profoundly impaired language*
        2. *If clinical picture is strongly suggestive of AS and FISH is negative, request 15q methylation study*
    E. *Rett's syndrome*
        1. *Classic phenotype is seen in females with autistic regression, microcephaly, seizures, and hand-wringing*
        2. *Males may present with Rett's syndrome, but presentation is varied; there is increased presentation of Rett's syndrome in males with Klinefelter's syndrome (47XXY)*
        3. *DNA test for MECP2 is positive in 80% of cases*
    F. *Smith–Lemli–Opitz syndrome*
        1. *Rare condition of cholesterol metabolism error*
        2. *Multiple congenital anomalies, failure to thrive, cognitive delay; occasional poly, syndactyly*
    G. *Fetal alcohol syndrome*
        1. *Maternal exposure to alcohol is worse in first trimester, but can yield significant impairment throughout pregnancy*
        2. *Exposure to alcohol carries a high risk for other substances of abuse*
        3. *Physical findings may be disproportionately subtle relative to cognitive and emotional issues*
  IX. *Autistic savant (see Chapter 13)*
    A. *Splintered exceptional skills in the context of significant social ± communication impairments*
    B. *Avoid exploitative settings*

(continued)

TABLE 5.1	Flowchart for Evaluation and Management of Autistic Spectrum Disorders (ASDs) Based on Presenting Symptoms *(continued)*

    C. *Behavior modification can maximize gifts and at the same time address communicative impairments*

    D. *Most commonly expressed in math, memory, musical, or artistic skills*

X. *Adults with an ASD (see Chapter 14)*

    A. *As patients, these individuals typically require extra time scheduled in an appointment to review with compulsive care issues regarding health care decisions*

    B. *The primary care provider (PCP) may wish to involve a psychologist to help individual explore best ways to maintain a balance between social withdrawal and social interaction*

    C. *Legal guidance is needed especially in situations where an adult with an ASD may need intermittent, regular part-time, or full-time assistance of other adults*

    D. *Avoid "warehousing"; independent living may not be optimal for socially vulnerable individuals, despite normal or near-normal cognition*

    E. *Individuals who have very mild ASD and very high functioning may need only cognitive counseling as issues with dating, career, marriage, and children arise*

XI. *Ethical considerations (see Chapter 15)*

    A. *Autonomy when possible*

        1. *Avoid warehousing whenever possible*

        2. *Important to respect the individual's need for privacy and still provide protection as needed, especially in areas of finance, relationships, sexuality, and bearing children*

        3. *Having a "safe place" to talk to a trusted counselor or mentor can be life saving*

        4. *Long-term goals may or may not include independent living, even for individuals with seemingly "mild" impairment*

    B. *Beneficence*

        1. *Maintain vigilance to neglect of health because of a seeming "oblivious" sense of need*

        2. *Actively working in the community to find best support systems for individuals with ASD is proactive and yields significant rewards for the PCP practice as well as individual*

    C. *Nonmaleficence*

        1. *Approach to sexuality should begin with education and when the individual is cognitively ready*

        2. *Reproduction rights should be measured by each individual, and in the "never competent" individual, a standard of best interest should be used, such that a cognitively impaired person who cannot provide self-care does not become pregnant*

    D. *Justice*

        1. *The active involvement of individuals with an ASD in a primary care practice helps provide needed care for a significant portion of the population who would not otherwise receive it*

    E. *Dignity always*

TABLE 5.2	Suggested Resources for Building the PCP-Centered Autism Team

1. *Social services: Can provide links to community resources for mental health; funding; coordination of many consultants working on behalf of one family*
2. *Behavioral developmental pediatrician: Pediatrician who is trained in abnormal behaviors, including Attention Deficit Hyperactivity Disorder (ADHD), learning disabilities (LD), and ASDs; is particularly adept at cognitively normal or near-normal children with abnormal behaviors*
3. *Pediatric psychiatrist: May or may not have the interest or ability to admit to inpatient psychiatric services; however, is instrumental in coordinating medications for rage, mood disorders, disorders of psychoses, and Tourette 's syndrome*
4. *Pediatric neurologist: Specializes in all aspects of abnormal neurologic problems in children, including delay, regression, epilepsy, and syndromic disorders*
5. *Neurodevelopmental disabilities pediatric neurologist: Specializes in all aspects of abnormal neurologic aspects of children, with particular interest in developmental disabilities. Typically have particular interest in autism, cognitive disorders, and traumatic brain injury survivors*
6. *Family law attorney: Essential for a family needing to plan long-term care for vulnerable child, particularly where state funding for life-time support may need to be identified and accessible for caregivers of the adult patients*
7. *Education specialist: Often not only has experience in most appropriate placement of a child in a given setting or school, but is adept in current federal and state laws pertaining to autism. In those children or teens who are high functioning and for whom college is an option, can be critically helpful in identifying best colleges. Also, can be very helpful in coaching families on how to navigate the public school and maximize the Admission, Review, and Dismissal (ARD) experience*
8. *Pediatric physical therapist (PT): Can provide clear guidelines for best outcome on frequency and types of PT, as well as recommendations for assistive devices*
9. *Pediatric occupational therapist: Helpful for identifying and treating a wide range of issues commonly associated with autism, including swallowing coordination problems; sensory and tactile defensiveness as well as neediness; dysgraphia; and may be able to recommend a variety of assistive technology as needed*
10. *Pediatric speech therapist: Those therapists who are particularly interested in receptive and expressive language as well as pragmatic and syntactic speech are usually able to provide very clear snapshots of a child's precise language needs, as well as make recommendations to schools as well as families regarding the frequency and types of therapies; may also be able to recommend speech-based assistive technologies*
11. *Assistive technology (AT) specialist: Typically associated with computer-based software, the use of AT can assist with communication and fine motor skills*
12. *Psychometrician: Whether private or through the public school, psychometricians are able to provide a wealth of data specific to cognition, attention, language, and math-based abilities*
13. *Counseling services: There is no substitute for a counselor who is willing and able to commit to the months to years that may be needed in ongoing support as an autistic child or teenager moves through the many phases of development in addition to his or her autism. Counseling services may need to include family and/or sibling therapy, as well as a range of counseling techniques, from play therapy, to behavior modification, to cognitive or "talk" therapy that is most salient to the client's needs*
14. *Autism educator: Whether private or public school employed, an educator with special training and interest in autism can be an invaluable resource to the pediatrician's office in streamlining requests. All schools require signed release from the parents before physicians can visit with the school; however, it is mutually beneficial when the school needs additional support or information from the physician in order to maximize services*
15. *Autism research team: Because there is such a drive to investigate causes and cures for autism, many excellent research teams exist all over the country. To access what research is happening in your region, or specific to the type of autism your patient may have, you may access http://www.nichd.nih.gov/autism/research/cpea.cfm?sortby=research*

SUGGESTED READINGS

Battaglia A, Bianchini E, Carey JC. Diagnostic yield of the comprehensive assessment of developmental delay/mental retardation in an institute of child neuropsychiatry. *Am J Med Genet.* 1999;82:60–66.

Fenichel GM. Psychomotor retardation and regression. In: *Clinical Pediatric Neurology: A Signs and Symptoms Approach.* 5th Ed. Philadelphia, PA: WB Saunders; 2005;117–147.

Frankenberg WE, Dodds JB. *The Denver Development Assessment (Denver II).* Denver, Colorado: The University of Colorado Medical School; 1992.

Shevell MI, Majnemer A, Rosenbaum P, Abrahamowicz M. Etiologic yield of subspecialists' evaluation of young children with global developmental delay. *J Pediatr.* 2000;136:593–598.

Shevell MI, Ashwal S, Donley D, et al. Neurology and The Practice Committee of the Child Neurology Society Report of the Quality Standards Subcommittee of the American Academy of Practice parameter: evaluation of the child with global developmental delay: *Neurology.* 2003;60;367–380. Retrieved June 13, 2010, from http://www.neurology.org/cgi/reprint/60/3/367.pdf

Shevell, MI, Swaimann, KF. Global developmental delay and mental retardation. In: *Pediatric Neurology: Principles and Practice.* 4th ed. St Louis, MO: Mosby; 551–560. 2006.

Thomason MJ, Lord J, Bain MD, et al. A systematic review of evidence for the appropriateness of neonatal screening programmes for inborn errors of metabolism. *J Public Health Med.* 1998;20:331–343.

Developmental Delays: Speech, Motor, Social, and Global

6

SAMPLE CASE

Elizabeth was 3 years old when her parents first brought her to the pediatrician for delay, stating that she only had a few words and no phrases. Additionally, she seemed exceptionally shy around other children, holding her ears when around a noisy group of children and seemingly preferring to play alone. She demonstrated some hand flapping when excited, but otherwise did not demonstrate a great deal of stereotypical behavior. Her history was significant for a healthy child born full term to a healthy first-time mother, and neither the child nor the mother had had any serious illnesses. She is an only child, and her parents who have recently immigrated from South Korea prefer to speak exclusively in their native language when at home. Her review of systems revealed no evidence for seizures, head trauma, or any other neurologic concerns. Further, there was no history on either side of the family for autism. A physical examination revealed a very shy child, but who, over a few minutes, gradually warmed to the examiner, would permit interaction with a variety of toys, and showed appropriate laughter and smiling with intermittent eye gaze. The rest of her examination was unremarkable. An audiology evaluation revealed no evidence of hearing loss. Serologic evaluations for routine chemistries were all normal. Psychometric testing revealed a normal cognitive profile, with delays in receptive language as well as adaptive skills of living, which manifested as anxiety. Although Elizabeth did not qualify for a diagnosis under the autism spectrum, she was able to receive services for delay in receptive and pragmatic speech, as well as delay in social skills. The family was encouraged to use both English and Korean at home. The child was placed with behavioral and speech therapies in an immersion classroom setting five mornings a week from 8 to 2 PM, and over the academic year, she made exceptional gains both in language and in socialization. At age 5, she is now enrolled in a mainstream public classroom setting, with ongoing speech support as needed.

MANAGING DEVELOPMENTAL DELAY AND AUTISTIC FEATURES

The most common complaint that prompts evaluation for autism is delay. Of all potential delays, the lag of expressive language is most readily identified by parents as a cause for concern (need cite). However, it is important for the primary care provider (PCP) to conscientiously evaluate motor, social, and cognitive parameters, as well as language (Table 6.1). Additionally, it is important for the PCP to appreciate the important difference between delay and regression.

Having parents reflect on the child's developmental progress while waiting for the appointment can be facilitated by having the parent complete a brief developmental screen prior to being called back to the examination room. Suggested single-page checklists are available in English, Spanish, and Mandarin in Appendix A at the back of this book. Having such a procedure in place for a primary care office makes assessing for development at every available chance and reduces the risk for missing subtle delays that otherwise may not be detected.

The slow acquisition of milestones may be due to either a static or progressive disorder. Static disorders are often seen in the context of structural lesions, from either injury, genetics, or perinatal insult. By contrast, progressive encephalopathies are more often associated with metabolic insults as well as neurocutaneous disorders (7). Regressive disorders refer to the loss of previously attained milestones and are discussed in a different chapter (3).

TABLE 6.1	Flowchart for Evaluation for Delay and Autistic Spectrum Disorders (1–3)

I. *Previsit (either sick or well)*
  A. *Parents complete developmental screen on arrival to office*
II. *History*
  A. *Perform Denver developmental screen II*
  B. *Review of any reported delay: verify slow (delayed) vs. loss of previously achieved skills (regression)*
  C. *Validate if newborn screening has been performed*
  D. *Perform careful family history, including risk for consanguinity or early postnatal deaths*
  E. *Perform careful perinatal history, with particular attention to gestation, birth weight, and any perinatal issues*
III. *Physical*
  A. *Observation of child with family and at play during history gathering*
  B. *Height, weight, and head circumference plotted and checked*
  C. *General examination with particular attention to possible dysmorphology; shape of spine, shape of head, skin lesions, and digits*
  D. *Eye contact, which needs to be specifically described as appropriate, fleeting, or none*
IV. *Laboratory evaluation*
  A. *Vision and auditory screening*
  B. *Fragile X with cognitive delay*
  C. *Urine organic acids, serum amino acids, and thyroid panels if no newborn screening*
  D. *EEG if presence of staring spells and/or convulsions*
  E. *If known familial or findings for specific disorder, specific test for that disorder*
  F. *If known historical or physical findings suggestive of central nervous system (CNS) injury or malformation, unenhanced MRI of head*
  G. *If known exposure to environmental lead, order lead screen*
  H. *If child has regressed, order comprehensive evaluation, including MRI, EEG, metabolic testing; cytogenetic screening; genetics consult; neurology consult*
V. *Specific findings*
  A. *Speech delay*
    1. *Speech assessment (may need to include specific request for expressive, receptive, pragmatic, and/or syntactic speech delay)*
    2. *Hearing assessment (may require a bilateral auditory evoked response)*
      a. *If delayed, consider MRI*
      b. *Lead levels*
    3. *Referral to assistive technology as indicated*
    4. *Consider referral for social skills coaching as indicated to facilitate pragmatic speech*
  B. *Social*
    1. *Psychometric testing*
      a. *Consider Vineland or other scale of adaptive behavior per public school or private diagnostician; may need additional psychometric measures for cognitive assessment*
      b. *May need play therapy as support for other speech or occupational therapy (OT)*
      c. *Mild-to-severe social impairment may be seen in individuals with Asperger's syndrome, but relatively sophisticated speech may mask symptoms initially*
    2. *Speech assessment: request specifically for receptive and pragmatic speech*
    3. *OT for sensory integration, for the child who seems particularly oblivious to his environment*
  C. *Motor*
    1. *OT assessment: can provide very specific snapshot of skills relative to age, with specific goal-driven therapy*
    2. *Physical therapy assessment*
    3. *Serologies: Creatine kinase (CK), especially prior to sedation for any investigation such as MRI*

TABLE 6.1	**Flowchart for Evaluation for Delay and Autistic Spectrum Disorders (1–3)** *(continued)*

D. *Cognitive*
   1. *Psychometric testing*
      a. *Have family request meeting with school officials to discuss results*
      b. *Family should aim for maintaining cordial relationships with school, but attempt to have thorough and explicit remedies implemented*
      c. *Advise family to keep copies of all school meetings and test results*
   2. *Serologies: fragile X; consider either genetic testing or referral; further metabolic assessment as driven by findings on physical examination*
   3. *Imaging: consider imaging if neurologic evaluation suggests focal findings in addition to cognitive delay, including but not limited to concerns of head size, shape, or dysmorphologies*

The hallmark of any evaluation for delay is one based on a careful, stratified approach as dictated by history and physical. Multiple screens are available for the practitioner within the context of a clinical visit, which can help clarify the degree to which a child may have delay either across the board or by language, social, gross, and fine motor skills. The Denver development assessment (DDST II) is one of several excellent skills that a PCP should be able to use quickly and reliably at all visits, because it does not rely on a child's cooperation in order to keep tabs on a child's ongoing development (1). Further, the American Academy of Neurology, in conjunction with the American Academy of Pediatrics, has provided guidelines on how PCPs should approach surveillance (5), and this can be accessed at http://www.neurology.org/cgi/reprint/60/3/367.pdf.

HISTORY

All visits with a child are opportunities to review development, even when the practitioner may be very busy. Having a family reflect on the child's development while waiting in the waiting room can help focus the family on any concerns that they may have. The history itself must provide five critically important points that will not come from any other aspect of the PCP's involvement with the family or child. By the end of the history gathering, the PCP should be able to identify if there is a static or progressive encephalopathy; the approximate developmental age of the child; the possible timing of the etiology, whatever that may be; the possibility of a genetic etiology; and finally the potential for rehabilitation for the child (6). If at the end of the history gathering, these items are not clear, it will be important to persist in obtaining additional medical records or interviewing other family members to clarify.

PHYSICAL

Unlike the luxury of examining adult patients, behavioral observations for children must be made throughout the interview. Hence, the physical examination for a child should actually start during the history, when the examiner can quietly observe how the child interacts with the family in a nonintrusive and nonthreatening manner, with toys, with the examiner in a playful and engaging manner. Having the weight, height, and head circumference accurately recorded and plotted on the appropriate growth chart and initialed by the PCP is an important way to not miss subtle changes in growth patterns. Additionally, the general examination should be performed, with particular attention to head shape, spine, skin lesions, or any dysmorphic features. Finally, if the child is walking, it is important for the PCP to evaluate his gait for any abnormalities.

LABORATORY TESTING

Although there is disagreement on the extent of metabolic testing for a child with delays, most authorities are in agreement that a careful, stratified approach is far more appropriate than a broad, shotgun approach that is typically very expensive with low yield (1,4–6).

- Visual assessment: any child with delay may need appropriate vision screening, which may or may not include a full ophthalmologic examination.
- Audiometric assessment: any child with delay, especially any evidence of social or speech delay, deserves an audiometric assessment, and may include behavioral audiometry or brain stem auditory evoked response testing when feasible.
- Consider metabolic screening and thyroid functions if there is no evidence that universal newborn screening has been done.
- Electroencephalogram (EEG) if there is history of suspicion of staring spells and/or convulsions.
- Consider referral to public school for psychometric assessment for in-depth intellectual and achievement scores if school age; for autism and/or speech and occupational assessment if below school age.

Once delay, for any and all parameters, have been identified, additional testing choices should be driven by findings.

LANGUAGE

Children who are referred for evaluation of autism most commonly present with either delayed language or loss of previously acquired language (Table 6.2). Further, the acquisition of language is the best correlate for long-term outcome, with those children who acquire no language by 5 years of age having the poorest outcome.

Autism is now conceptualized as a behavioral phenotype that occurs from many different etiologies. Infantile autism presents with failure of language development, severe impairment of interpersonal relationships, a restricted repertoire of activities, and onset before 3 years. Indeed the most common complaint from a family may be the delay of onset of language or the loss of a few words that had been previously acquired.

All children who present with language delay must have auditory evaluations that screen specifically for both expressive and receptive language functions. Mental retardation, or cognitive delay, is by far the most common cause of language delay, and at 3% of all children, it is far more common than autism. More than 80% of these children have mild cognitive delay, with full-scale intelligence quotient (IQ) between 50% to 70%. Developmental language disorders may

TABLE 6.2	Differential Diagnosis for Language Delay
Cognitive delay	
Developmental language disorders	
Autism	
Acquired language disorders	
Hearing loss	
Dysarthria	
Muscular dystrophies	
Acquired epileptiform aphasia	

also mask as cognitive delay, in which children struggle with the conversational aspect of communication. Subsequently, any child with a language disorder must have an exhaustive speech evaluation that is sensitive to not only expressive and receptive language, but pragmatic and semantic speech as well. Autistic spectrum disorders are characterized by speech delays; however, it is important to note that individuals with Asperger's syndrome have a normal onset of expressive speech, but the content is often unusual in its content. Indeed, individuals with Asperger's syndrome may score very high on verbal portions of achievement tests, but quite low on performance and nonverbal skills.

Clearly all children with language delay deserve a complete hearing screen, because it is critical to the management of not only the child's language acquisition but all other aspects of the child's life. Hearing loss may be genetic or not, may be total or subtotal, may be unilateral or bilateral, but all forms will profoundly affect the child's development.

Selective mutism has been seen in children who suffered trauma, but this is typically discovered from history with a clear event with subsequent loss of language, and is a diagnosis by exclusion only. In such children, typically normal hearing screens can be obtained, and the child may need referral to child psychiatry or counseling.

Of note, because children with Duchenne's as well as Becker's muscular dystrophy may present with social and cognitive delays, it is important to request a serum CK level before ordering a magnetic resonance imaging (MRI), in which general sedation may be used, because of inherent risk for cardiac function.

SOCIALIZATION

In children who are referred for delay in socialization, it is important to note that social skills need not be absent or even egregiously abnormal to warrant concern and further evaluation. In the examination room, the practitioner should be able to take note of the child's capacity for eye contact, whether it is fleeting, absent, or intermittent. Shy children may not wish to immediately warm to a practitioner, but the quality of maintaining eye contact should be investigated by both history and physical examination. It is also important to realize that even children with autism are capable of sustaining eye contact with close family members. Therefore, it still merits concern when a child can maintain eye contact, but with only one or two close family members. In addition to poor eye contact, the family may report and the examiner may be able to observe oddness in body posture, facial expressions, and other critically important nonverbal skills appropriate to age.

For children who are seemingly much more immature relative to age, but who do not truly exhibit oddities in behavior, additional environmental factors may need to be concerned relative to exposure to other children on a consistent basis for adequate development of social skills, versus stressors at home such as single parents who are juggling with several jobs and/or school.

Finally, some children may exhibit symptoms consistent with impulse control problems from a variety of etiologies, including but not limited to attention deficit hyperactivity disorder, mood disorders, oppositional defiant disorders, cognitive delay, and adjustment disorders (Table 6.3). Careful attention to history and physical should help elicit important clues in this regard, and confirmation is obtained by psychometric assessment, either through the public school or through private testing.

Of note, because children with Duchenne's as well as Becker's muscular dystrophy may present with social and cognitive delays, it is important to request a serum CK level before ordering an MRI, in which general sedation may be used, because of inherent risk for cardiac function.

FINE MOTOR SKILLS

Children who struggle with tasks requiring dexterity typically require a symptom-based approach for diagnosis and management. Although fine motor delay may appear early on, the most common referral for fine motor delay is dysgraphia for children who demonstrate difficulty and easy fatiguing while gripping a pen or pencil. Nevertheless, increasing recognition has come about in the last decade with regard to some children who seem particularly sensory defensive or sensory

TABLE 6.3	Differential Diagnoses for Socialization Delay

Inadequate opportunity for socialization

Immaturity

Attention deficit disorders

Oppositional defiant disorders

Autism

Muscular dystrophies

Chronic illness

One or more nonnative languages spoken at home

Shyness

needy, or have a combination of both. The result is often awkwardness in how a child approaches fine motor tasks.

The astute PCP may be able to reduce the severity of these behaviors by being particularly observant of the child in infancy and preschool years. Children should ordinarily be able to bring both hands to midline by 10 months, clap by 12 months, deliberately release items by 12 months, use a fisted grip for crayons by 18 months, and use scissors by 30 months. Other concerning signs included drooling during tasks that involve intense concentration, using only one hand to complete tasks always, or not being able to open one hand.

Early referral to a pediatric occupational therapist, with specific concerns noted on the referral form (e.g., appears to keep left hand fisted most of the time) can be a critically important step in the identification of any other potential delays, as well as provide remediation and rehabilitation for the child.

GROSS MOTOR SKILLS

Children with delayed gross motor development have a wide range of potential differential diagnoses (Table 6.4), and must be approached with a systematic approach to evaluation. In the

TABLE 6.4	Differential Diagnosis for Motor Delay

Hypotonia
    Cerebral hypotonia
    Spinal cord disorders
    Spinal muscular atrophies
    Polyneuropathies
    Disorders of neuromuscular transmissions
    Metabolic and fiber-type disproportion myopathies
    Myositis
    Muscular dystrophies

Hypertonia
    Cerebral palsy
    Stroke
    Demyelinating disease
    Brain abscess
    Sturge Weber
    Familial syndromes

absence of language and social delay, the child with gross motor delay is often hypotonic and may have a neuromuscular disease (4). The exhaustive evaluation of motor dysfunction is beyond the scope of this text; however, clues to the origin of weakness may be made from the degree of tone, the distribution of weakness, and the careful examination of reflexes.

Certainly any history that suggests intrapartum asphyxia should prompt head imaging. Also, any physical findings that suggest dysmorphic features, abnormally shaped skull, neurocutaneous lesions, or structural abnormalities should prompt the request for an unenhanced MRI of the head. If general sedation is required for the MRI, a screen for serum creatine kinase (CK) should be ordered to rule out early presentation of a muscular dystrophy (MD), because children with MD do not tolerate general anesthesia.

Additionally, any child with gross motor delay deserves an immediate referral to both a pediatric and occupational therapist for a thorough assessment, as well as recommendations for rehabilitation and remediation.

SUMMARY

The most common cause for referral for autism is concern for delay in either one or more parameters, most notably communication and socialization. However, children with autistic features may present with a wide range of delays that also include gross and fine motor delays. The astute PCP, whose time is limited with a family whether for a sick or well check, has the family fill out a development assessment sheet on arrival to the office in order to help focus the parent's attention on any developmental concerns at hand. The PCP then takes advantage of the history not only to garner precisely where the child is developmentally, but to observe the child in an nonintrusive way for important behavioral clues. Finally, if concerns exist for developmental delays, referrals for vision and hearing screens are made, as well as any other laboratory assessment that the history and physical may dictate. Ultimately, referrals to other specialists may be made at that same visit if concern exists about genetic, epileptic, or neurologic issues that are beyond the scope of the PCP's office.

REFERENCES

1. Frankenberg WE, Dodds JB. *The Denver Development Assessment (Denver II)*. Denver, Colorado: The University of Colorado Medical School; 1992.
2. Shevell MI, Majnemer A, Rosenbaum P, Abrahamowicz M. Etiologic yield of subspecialists' evaluation of young children with global developmental delay. *J Pediatr.* 2000;136:593–598.
3. Battaglia A, Bianchini E, Carey JC. Diagnostic yield of the comprehensive assessment of developmental delay/mental retardation in an institute of child neuropsychiatry. *Am J Med Genet.* 1999;82:60–66.
4. Fenichel GM. Psychomotor retardation and regression. In: *Clinical Pediatric Neurology: A Signs and Symptoms Approach*. Philadelphia, PA: WB Saunders; 2005;117–147.
5. Shevell MI, Ashwal S, Donley D, et al. Neurology and the Practice Committee of the Child Neurology Society Report of the Quality Standards Subcommittee of the American Academy of Practice parameter: evaluation of the child with global developmental delay. *Neurology.* 2003;60;367–380. Retrieved June 13, 2010, from http://www.neurology.org/cgi/reprint/60/3/367.pdf
6. Shevell MI, Swaimann, KF. Global developmental delay and mental retardation. In: Swaimann KF, Ashwal S, eds. *Pediatric Neurology: Principles and Practice*. 4th ed. St Louis, MO: Mosby;2006; 551–560.
7. Stromme P, Kanavin OJ, Abdelnoor M, Woldseth B, Rootwelt T, Diderichsen J, Bjurulf B, Sommer F, Magnus P. Incidence rates of progressive childhood encephalopathy in Oslo, Norway: a population based study. *BMC Pediatr* 2007;7:25. Retrieved November 4, 2010 from EBSCOhost.

7 Odd Behaviors

SAMPLE CASE

No one wanted to be around Bradley, a 7-year-old highly verbal boy who seemed very impulsive and distractible. The last straw was when at a music class Bradley became bored and began licking the soles of his shoes. At that point, the mother brought the child to the office and began describing a long litany of odd sensory and motor behaviors, including headbanging and eyelash plucking. Indeed, he had managed to remove two sets of eyelashes in the last 2 years. At that time, he was being served through the public school for Attention Deficit Hyperactivity Disorder (ADHD) combined. However, the subsequent emergence of odd behaviors, particularly in social settings, prompted concern for possibly high-functioning autistic spectrum disorder (ASD). Psychometric testing revealed that Bradley most closely fit an Asperger's syndrome, with general anxiety. The addition of aripiprazole significantly reduced the anxiety and poor boundary issues. Occupational therapy (OT) was instituted to reduce sensory neediness, which including skin brushing, joint compression, and weighted vests. Finally, the addition of a behavior-modification program instituted across all environments at both home and school provided needed structure for reducing unwanted behaviors.

MANAGING ODD BEHAVIORS

One of the hallmarks of the behavioral phenotype of ASDs includes the presentation of odd behaviors, which include self-injury, social inappropriateness, obsession and rituals, sexual inappropriateness, and odd sensory behaviors.

Self-Injurious Behavior

Of all the worrisome behaviors that individuals with ASD demonstrate, the issue of self-injury is perhaps the most upsetting for all involved. In the most severe cases, self-injurious behavior (SIB) can result in retinal detachment, blindness, broken bones, bleeding, or death (1). SIB is displayed by 10% to 15% of individuals with autism and intellectual disabilities. These estimates are higher among individuals living in institutions and among those with greater cognitive impairments. Individuals with ASD typically self-abuse by one of three basic forms: headbanging, biting, or scratching. Typically precipitated by frustration, a child or adult with ASD may have eruptions of these behaviors that develop into more ritualistic patterns long after the initial upset has passed.

Typically the precipitating event is based on an environmental upset: the child has a preferred toy removed, a change in routine, or encounters a highly stimulating environment. Less often a child is simply bored and seeking the attention of adults around him. Rarely does increase in self-injury reflect an acute illness, but this must be considered in a child who might be prone to urinary tract, sinus, or ear infections, especially in the absence of fever and the inability to articulate what hurts. In addition to attention seeking and relief of frustration, some research suggests that SIB may result in the release of chemicals in the brain that produce pleasurable effects. Although there is considerable evidence to support of all these explanations, current thought indicates that SIB is a highly complex, heterogeneous phenomenon that is often attributable to a combination of factors.

Prevention of the behavior is key, because over time, SIB reinforces its power to caregivers to attend immediately to the individual with an attempt to reduce the injury often by acquiescing to demands, whether appropriate or not.

The use of helmets can help defer frontal bossing, as well as the development of cauliflower ear, both of which are acquired deformities from repeated blows but apart from the cosmetic appearance, represent no true injury. However, many individuals resist wearing them because of discomfort and heat, or simply because sensory issues may prohibit the individual from ever being comfortable with wearing a helmet. Further, adjusting medication for aggression or anxiety may also help reduce self-injury. The primary care provide (PCP) may wish to consider starting with an atypical antipsychotic if there is any concern that using a selective serotonin reuptake inhibitor (SSRI) may aggravate existing aggression because of the activating qualities of many SSRIs. Caregivers should always seek ways to anticipate the behaviors by being aware of what environmental triggers are most upsetting. Finally caregivers need to be alert for any evidence of the underlying illness such as an occult infection or injury (1–3).

Social Inappropriateness

More common than SID, social inappropriateness is found in virtually all individuals with an ASD. The social awkwardness ranges from being mildly inconsiderate of other's statements or feelings to literally staring through family members and caregivers as though invisible. Social issues are highly individual and largely dependent on cognitive strengths and weaknesses, as well as the family's capacity to cope with challenging behavior.

For reasons still not well understood, the individual with an ASD does not conform to the conventional need to interact with others. People with an ASD may be perceived as being "rude" or odd. Behaviors may include staring, walking through conversations, walking over people, and disregard of other social expectations of society. Subsequently, individuals with ASD may be isolated even further not only because of their behaviors, but because of their seeming lack of understanding or empathy that there is a problem.

For all such individuals, it is imperative that in addition to the standard evaluation that all individuals receive for etiology of their autistic behaviors, they receive social skills coaching. Particularly high-functioning individuals, as they mature into the teenage years, have strong motivation to blend in socially and coaching, and can find ways to enter into conversations more easily (4–6).

Obsession and Ritual

According to the diagnostic criteria for autism, repetitive and stereotyped behavior demonstrating restricted interests and activities is a basic expression of the condition. Children with autism may seem to be puzzling obsessed with some nonfunctional object or part of a toy and may become very disturbed when it is taken away from them. Indeed, the oddest aspect may be that the object or toy is being used for functions for which it was not designed, such as the doll used as a hammer or the sets of toy cars as devices to systematically throw at some perceived target. Other obsessions may include an in-depth knowledge about a very narrow topic, such as flags of foreign countries; the in-depth knowledge of a prehistoric age, schedules for trains and buses, or math calculations and dates. Apart from obsession with items that require an in-depth database, many individuals with an ASD are also obsessed with routine, specifically in the schedule of the day, the arrangement of furniture in home and school, and even the route in which a caregiver may drive the individual to and from school or work.

As in many individuals with a compulsive–obsessive disorder, the goal of therapy is determined by the degree of dysfunction the obsession renders in daily life. It is important to recognize the importance of these behaviors and the role they play in the everyday lives of people with autism. Routine is a means by which they understand and feel safe within our environment. It makes the world reliable and predictable.

However, routine may not always be able to be followed, and access to the object of obsession may not always be available to the individual. In such cases, the PCP may be asked to assist in medication and therapeutic options to help relieve the panic or rage that ensues in order to allow the home to be functional. Most individuals are helped by ongoing behavior-modification therapy that is either a routine part of an individual's day, especially for younger children and teenagers in the public, or a private classroom. However, an adult may need behavior modification therapy as well, with goal-specific therapies directed at how to best self-soothe when the compulsion becomes intolerable.

Additionally, the PCP may wish to evaluate the need to add specific medication for the relief of the most troublesome aspects of the obsessive behaviors. This may mean adding a low dose of an SSRI to reduce the overall anxiety. Alternatively, if the SSRI is at risk for activating negative or aggressive behaviors, the use of an atypical antipsychotic, such as risperidone or aripiprazole, may be appropriate (1–3,6).

Stereotypical Behavior

Along the lines of obsession and ritual, it is important to recognize stereotypical behavior as a separate entity. Stereotypical behavior refers specifically to either simple or complex motor and vocal activities that are repetitive and serves to provide immediate relief for the momentary anxiety, upset, or anger an individual may have (Table 7.1). Whatever the source of interest or the area of routine, stereotypes serve important roles to individuals with an ASD. At least some literature suggests that the role of spinning, for example, is comforting in removing the overwhelming amount of stimulus an individual with ASD is confronting, and serves to minimize background intrusion (3). It is perhaps inevitable that when these obsessions, rituals, or stereotypies are disrupted, the response may be likely extreme and excessive, especially where there is no clearly understood reason for the interruption. The combination of adequate transition preparation, associated with behavior modification and medication as necessary, can provide significant relief to individuals whose behaviors significantly interrupt their day and activities.

Sexual Inappropriateness

Inappropriate sexual behaviors are a subset of challenging behaviors that may directly affect the integration of individuals with ASDs. Researchers are exploring how to limit the stigmatizing

TABLE 7.1	Examples of Stereotypical Behavior in ASD
Simple motor	*Repetitive headbanging, flicking fingers, rolling objects, pulling on pieces of string, spinning objects or staring at objects that spin; tapping and scratching, inspecting, walking along and tracing lines and angles; feeling particular textures, cloths, etc.; rocking, standing up, and jumping; tapping, scratching, or manipulating other parts of the body; repetitive headbanging or self-injury; teeth grinding, sexual gratification*
Complex motor	*Intense attachment to particular objects for no apparent reason, such as cameras, DVD players, or other mechanical items; fascination with regular repeated patterns of objects or sounds; repetitively arranging, often in very precise patterns, toys or similar objects; collection of large numbers of unusual items, such as plastic bottles, rocks, paper clips, for no apparent reason*
Simple vocal	*Repetitive grunting, screaming, or making of other noises*
Complex vocal	*Fascination with certain complex topics, such as dinosaurs, television schedules, demands that statements from caregivers be erased using the sound of a DVD going in reverse; repetitively asking the same complex questions and demanding extensive and careful responses each time*
Complex routines	*Insistence on identical routes to certain places and at identical time; lengthy and complex rituals for showers, baths, or bedtimes; repetition of complex motor movements performed in a precise manner, such as genuflection or hand and arm gestures*

effect of problematic sexual behavior, and efforts are now directed at using language that avoids those which suggest sexual offending and abuse, and moving to language that implicitly embraces the normal sexual development in individuals with learning disorders. Terms such as "sexualized challenging behavior" or "sexual inappropriateness" are usually more applicable in individuals whose communication and socialization skills are innately impaired, but for whom there is no evidence for true criminal behavior (7). Typically sexual inappropriateness for individuals with autism involve self- and other-directed behaviors related to touch, exposure, and communication, which many educators, therapists, and clinicians view as distinct from sexual offending. As such, the subject of sexual maturation and behaviors is worthy of a separate discussion apart from other inappropriate behaviors.

Individuals with an ASD experience sexuality as other children, who may also fondle themselves particularly during early childhood. Although sexual awareness and urges are normal, the additional issues of social unawareness coupled with a propensity for anxiety may create extra temptation for an individual with an ASD to either attempt to fondle self or others, or to use language that is not appropriate. The following issues, while no means exhaustive, to be addressed in this chapter include inappropriate touching and masturbation, sexually risky behavior, and social issues surrounding romance and dating as teenagers and adults.

Masturbating

Masturbation is an issue that can present behavior problems at all ages. At times, masturbation may take on a near-compulsive quality for individuals with autism. For caregivers, finding ways to redirect behavior can be challenging. Low-functioning individuals for whom there is limited verbal understanding may respond best with simply redirecting and behavioral rewards for limiting self-touching in public areas, with restraints to private settings. Failing behavioral redirection and refocusing on other objects, individuals with an ASD may benefit from the use of behavioral medications that are directed to reducing anxiety or aggression. For individuals who compulsively masturbate and for whom genuine efforts at minimizing environmental stress and redirection have failed, the PCP may wish to consider the use of either SSRIs or atypical antipsychotic medication. As always, the PCP must be alert to the possibility of activating qualities of SSRIs, and in individuals who may already be aggressive, may wish to consider the use of an atypical antipsychotic in its place (2). For higher functioning and verbal individuals, the use of environmental rewards and behavior modification, with nonjudgmental redirection to self-handle only in private is usually sufficient. However, even for high-functioning verbal individuals, sometimes anxiety can be overwhelming and the temptation to masturbate is difficult. In such cases, again, a low dose of either an SSRI or an atypical antipsychotic may be helpful.

Risky Sexual Behavior

All individuals with impaired social understanding are at risk to be exploited sexually. To this end, it is very important to recognize that most postpubertal individuals with an ASD are capable of fertility. Although ethical questions about the appropriateness of practicing birth control need to be assessed for each individual, all parents and PCPs must review expectations, risks, and strategies to minimize the risk for an unwanted pregnancy for an individual with an ASD. Additionally, most strategies for minimizing pregnancies, short of abstinence, will not protect adequately against sexually transmitted illnesses. If the need for sexually driven behavior is truly more a sign of compulsivity rather than normal exploratory behavior, it may be necessary to carefully review the environment and possible risk factors, as well as consider the use of either an SSRI or an atypical antipsychotic to help reduce compulsivities and anxieties.

Romance and Dating

One of the great thought leaders about integrating individuals with ASDs into mainstream society, Dr. Temple Grandin has written numerous and excellent texts on the challenges faced by individuals with an ASD for the complexities of social settings, but also for romance and dating (8–11). Dr. Grandin, herself diagnosed with autism at a young age, has been a champion for broad social inclusion of individuals with an ASD diagnosis. Individuals with an ASD who are contemplating dating and marriage possibly benefit from both cognitive counseling to identify possible problem areas in social skills and medication as needed to reduce impulsivity and compulsivity when practicing intimacy. Certainly, the goal for any individual with a communication or social impairment is to provide the individual with all the skills necessary to have the independence to choose whether or not he or she wishes to date, become intimate, marry, and have children. Whether the individual chooses any or all of these options should ideally be at the individual's discretion, but not because of lack of skills or understanding on how to proceed (8–11).

Odd Sensory Seeking and Defensiveness

Perhaps one of the most puzzling symptoms that many individuals with ASD exhibit, especially as children, is either the repulsion of normal stimuli or, by contrast, the unusual attraction to ordinarily off-putting stimuli. Those individuals who appear to smell, taste, touch, and handle many different objects, including unusual items, are sometimes said to be "sensory needy." By contrast, those individuals who reject a wide range of items, including objects or sensations that are typically desirable or pleasant, are sometimes said to be "sensory defensive." Most individuals with an ASD who present with sensory issues often have both qualities. Indeed, at times, it can be difficult to sort out which sensory issues, the defensiveness or the neediness, need attention first.

The term "sensory integration disorder" (SID) has come into the literature, but is not a term found in the *DSM-IV*. Controversy still exists on what truly defines SID and what mechanisms for remediation are best. Evidence for both top-down (cognitive) and bottom-up (subcortical) causes for sensory and perceptual deficits has been sought (12). It has been suggested that the rare individuals who qualify as autistic savants are in fact the best example of the multimodal aberrant sensory function in autism (13).

The role of OT cannot be overemphasized for these individuals, and without doubt, the younger an individual is when OT is initiated for the relief of sensory issues, the far better the outcome. However, OT may be critically helpful at any point in the life span, and should be recommended to the family for those children who seem to be either tactilely needy or defensive. Occupational therapists can offer a wide range of sensory therapies that may range from skin brushing and joint compression to having a child swing on a platform and attempt to throw beanbags at a stable target. Indeed, the routine use of OT for children with sensory issues has been found to be fundamentally helpful in allowing other therapies, such as speech and social skills coaching, and academics proceed more successfully (14,15). Speech therapy may also be indicated if most of the sensory problems arise from either a sensitivity to the mouth area defensively (refuses to eat certain textures of food) or a tendency to orally explore odd or offensive items (2,14–16). Although the arena for therapies related to minimizing sensory issues is quite broad, it is a field in need of much more controlled and peer-reviewed research. For instance, anecdotal reports exist on the benefits of horseback riding or "equine" therapies (17,18); however, the access to specialty equine centers, quite apart from the cost, is typically neither practical nor an option for most families. Without more evidence-based research to carefully assess its role in individuals with autism, equine therapies are not recommended.

A great deal more peer-reviewed and evidence-based work is needed to better understand which modalities of occupational, social, and speech therapies are best suited for specific sensory issues with an ASD. However, early studies do support the role of goal-directed occupational therapies, and at times, speech and behavior therapies, for many sensory problems seen in ASD. As with any issue in autism, the therapy must be judiciously chosen and crafted to be part of a holistic approach to each individual.

SUMMARY

There is a movement among some individuals with higher functioning autism and Asperger's diagnoses to avoid changing individuals from their native Asperger's state into something "they are not," which is a nonautistic individual (8). Certainly, an individual's autonomy is to be

TABLE 7.2	Flowchart for ASD and Odd Behaviors

I. *Sensory defensiveness/neediness*
   A. *Refer to OT for assessment*
   B. *Consider speech therapy if sensory issues revolve around feeding or oral motor problems*
   C. *No or insufficient improvement; consider either an SSRI or an antipsychotic for exceptional problems*

II. *Social awkwardness*
   A. *Refer to behavioral modification; consider cognitive therapy and/or virtual reality therapy for individuals with verbal, high-functioning, or Asperger's syndrome*
      1. *No or insufficient improvement; consider anxiolytic for exceptional problems*

III. *Obsession and ritual*
   A. *Provide stable and predictable environment and routine*
   B. *Consider use of OT to coach self-soothing techniques, often in conjunction with behavioral therapy*
      1. *No or insufficient improvement; consider either an SSRI or an antipsychotic for exceptional problems*

IV. *Stereotypical behavior*
   A. *Provide stable and predictable environment and routine*
   B. *Consider use of OT to assist with redirection and refocusing if stereotypies are self-abusing or interfering with daily functioning*
      1. *No or insufficient improvement; consider either an SSRI or an antipsychotic for exceptional problems*

V. *Self-abusing behavior*
   A. *Provide stable and predictable environment and routine*
   B. *Consider what provocations are particularly troublesome, and attempt to remove or change if possible*
   C. *Consider physical therapy consult for physical supports, such as helmets, arm splints, etc., to minimize harm*
   D. *Consider OT to find substitute items for self-soothing*
      1. *No or insufficient improvement; consider either an SSRI or an antipsychotic for exceptional problems*

respected as much as possible, and ideally to be limited only by an individual's capacity for self-care and understanding (19). The goal of any therapies directed to the wide range of troublesome behavior in this chapter (Table 7.2) is first and foremost for the benefit of the individual with an ASD. Ideally individuals become autonomous enough to decide if they wish to participate in any particular social gathering or function. However, it is important that individuals have the necessary social tools coached and available to them so that the individual with ASD may elect to chose whether he or she wishes to be part of any particular group. Having the ability to choose, with the skills to participate if desired, is critical to the ethical care for any individual with a disability, and certainly applies to those individuals who must navigate complex social settings in the context of their own ASD.

REFERENCES

1. Thompson T. (2010). Self-injury in autism. Retrieved June 21, 2010, from http://travis-thompson.net/#/self-injury/4518767773
2. Myers SM, Johnson CP. Management of children with autism spectrum disorders. *Pediatrics*. 2007;5 (120): 1162–1182. http://aappolicy.aappublications.org/cgi/content/full/pediatrics%3B120/5/1162
3. Nadel J, Croue S, Mattlinger, M-J, et al. Do children with autism have expectancies about the social behaviour of unfamiliar people? A pilot study using the still face paradigm. *Autism Int J Res Pract*. 2000;4:133–146.

4. Downs A, Smith T. Emotional understanding, cooperation, and social behavior in high-functioning children with autism. *J Autism Dev Disord*. 2004;34:625–635.

5. Graetz JE, Spampinato K. Asperger's syndrome and the voyage through high school: not the final frontier. *J Coll Admission*. 2008;198:19–24

6. Matson JL, Dempsey T. The nature and treatment of compulsions, *obsessions*, and rituals in people with developmental disabilities. *Res Dev Disabil*. 2009;30:603–611.

7. Lockhart K, Guerin S, Shanahan S, Coyle K. Defining "sexualized challenging behavior" in adults with intellectual disabilities. *J Policy Pract Intellect Disabil*. 2009;6:293–301.

8. Grandin T, Barron S. *Unwritten Rules of Social Relationships: Decoding Social Mysteries through the Unique Perspectives of Autism*. Arlington, TX: Future Horizons; 2005. Retrieved November 4th, 2010 from http://www.templegrandin.com/templegrandinbooks.html

9. Baker J. *Preparing for Life: The Complete Guide for Transitioning to Adulthood for Those with Autism and Asperger's Syndrome*. Arlington, TX: Future Horizons; 2006.

10. Grandin T. *The Way I See It*. Arlington, TX: Future Horizons; 2008. Retrieved November 4th, 2010 from http://www.templegrandin.com/templegrandinbooks.html

11. Grandin T. *Emergence: My Life with Autism*. Novato, CA: Arena Press; 1986. Retrieved November 4th from http://www.templegrandin.com/templegrandinbooks.html

12. Rapin I. Atypical sensory/perceptual responsiveness. In: Tuchman R, Rapin I, eds. *Autism: A Neurological Disorder of Early Brian Development*. London: MacKeith Press; 2006:202–230.

13. Treffert DA. The savant syndrome in autistic disorder. In: Casanova MF, ed. *Recent Developments in Autism Research*. New York: Nova Science; 2005. 27–55.

14. Foss-Feig JH, Kwakye, LD, Cascio, CJ, et al. An extended multisensory temporal binding window in *autism* spectrum disorders. *Exp Brain Res*. 2010;203:381–389.

15. Fitzer A, Sturmey P. *Language and Autism*: *Applied Behavior Analysis, Evidence, and Practice*. Austin, TX: Pro-Ed, Inc; 2009.

16. Kim K, Disare K, Pfeiffer M, Kerker BD, McVeigh KH. Effects of individual and neighborhood characteristics on the timeliness of provider designation for early intervention services in New York City. *J Dev Behav Pediatr*. 2009;30:38–49.

17. Wuang Y, Wang C, Huang M, Su C. The effectiveness of simulated developmental horse-riding program in children with *autism*. *Adapt Phys Activ Q*. 2010;27:113–126.

18. de Reure A, Lorin A. Autistic children in pony therapy: evaluation scales and psychological and ethological approaches concerning relational, emotional and communication fields. *Neuropsychiatrie de l'Enfance et de l'Adolescence*. 2009;57:275–286.

19. Barnbaum DR. *The Ethics of Autism: Among Them, but Not of Them. Bioethics and the Humanities*. Indianapolis, IN: Indiana University Press; 2008.

Autistic Spectrum Disorders and Regression

SAMPLE CASE

Angela is a beautiful 4-year-old girl who is brought to the office with her parents, who state that although she had been on time for all motor, social, and communication milestones the first 18 months of life, after that time she stopped learning any new skills. Indeed, after that time, she lost the few words she had, as well as any socialization that she had had even at 6 months of age. Her parents reported that she now seemed preoccupied with spinning, finger flicking, hand flapping, and significantly worse tantrums than she had had as a toddler.

Physical examination revealed a bright child whose gaze was fleeting and who was difficult to redirect. However, the examination was essentially normal with no evidence for either general or neurologic findings. A Denver Developmental Screening Test II (DDST II) revealed a significant delay in communication and social skills not greater than 6 months each, but with preserved gross and fine motor skills as appropriate for age. Laboratory investigation revealed no abnormalities, including normal hearing and vision screens; normal electroencephalogram (EEG); normal magnetic resonance imaging (MRI) of head; negative fragile X, normal XY karyotype, normal liver and thyroid functions, serum amino acid, complete blood count (CBC) with differential, lactate, pyruvate, carnitine; with normal levels for urine organic acids.

The child was then started with speech therapy and occupational therapy through the local public school. The family did not have sufficient funding to pursue private therapies, so applied behavioral analysis (ABA) was not affordable, nor was it offered through the local public school system. Resources were provided to the family to implement environmental changes to create a more predictable setting both at home and at school. Names of family therapists were provided as well for family counseling, with specific concern directed at the slightly older siblings who were frequently frustrated with and embarrassed by Angela's odd behaviors. Finally, behavior modification therapists through the schools were consulted to help the family target the most worrisome behaviors, specifically tantrums, to better handle Angela's tantrums. No medications were indicated at this time.

MANAGEMENT OF REGRESSIVE BEHAVIOR

When exactly does autistic regression occur and what does it look like? Research indicates that the mean age of regression is at 27 months and that the regression itself seems to occur over a relatively quick space of time, usually 3 months with particularly pronounced regression in communication and social behavior (1,2). However, although communication and social behavior are most pronounced in autistic regression, other skills may also be affected, including motor coordination, sensory issues, and self-soothing, which may present as odd behaviors, including self-injury and exceptional anger. Further, the emergence of seizures may also be seen. Finally, aberrant head circumference, particularly in the first year of life, appears to be more often seen in children who regress and develop autistic features.

AUTISTIC REGRESSION WITH EPILEPSY, COGNITIVE DECLINE, AND SLEEP DISORDERS

Autistic regression is often associated with the overlap of at least two issues, including the emergence of epilepsy as well as loss of cognitive function (3,4). Perhaps the most researched of these factors to date are epilepsy and persons with intellectual disabilities, which overlap at high rates in persons with autistic regression (4). Additionally, significant overlap occurs in the context of autistic regression and cognitive regression: one study found more than 90% individuals with autistic regression from had an IQ less than 70. Still others have identified the emergence of sleep disturbances accompanying the issue of autistic regression as well. (5,6).

The definition, etiology, and diagnostic methodology for the study of ASD has grown and changed rapidly (Table 8.1). Research has emerged focusing on autistic regression and its

---

TABLE 8.1	Flowchart for Regression and ASDs

I. *Previously developmentally appropriate child now regressing with autistic features*
  A. *Neurophysiology*
    1. *All children with regression*
      a. *Routine EEG*
        1. *Abnormal: refer to pediatric neurology for management*
        2. *Normal: consider overnight or extended EEG tracing*
      b. *Overnight EEG*
        1. *Abnormal: refer to pediatric neurology*
        2. *Normal: monitor clinically*
      c. *Hearing screen*
      d. *Vision screen*
    2. *Both cognitive and motor decline with elevated serum creatine kinase*
      a. *Nerve conduction/motor conduction studies*
      b. *Referral to pediatric neuromuscular specialist*
      c. *Referral to genetics*
  B. *Imaging: MRI without contrast of head*
    1. *Normocephalic*
      a. *Abnormal: consider referral to pediatric neurology and genetics*
      b. *Normal: repeat only if clinical examination changes*
    2. *Macrocephalic*
      a. *Hydrocephalus: consider referral to pediatric neurosurgery*
      b. *Normal or atrophic: Alexander and Canavan*
  C. *Serologies*
    1. *Isolated decline of cognitive function*
      a. *Urine organic acids: galactosemia, Sanfilippo, and maple syrup urine*
        1. *Disease; homocystinuria*
      b. *Serum amino acid: histidinemia and homocysteinemia*
      c. *Serum chemistries: creatine kinase, liver function, and CBC with differential, lactate, pyruvate, and carnitine*
      d. *Genetic screens: fragile X, chromosome analysis and DNA microarray*
    2. *Coarse facial features*
      a. *Thyroid function*
        1. *Hypothyroidism: refer to pediatric endocrinology*
        2. *Euthyroid: Hurler phenotype: evaluate for mucopolysaccharidoses*
    3. *Motor decline*
      a. *Creatine kinase: if elevated, refer to pediatric neurology*
    4. *Skin changes:*
      a. *Genetic evaluation as indicated for neurofibromatosis and tuberous*
        1. *Sclerosis or other neurocutaneous disorders*
    5. *HIV risk*
      a. *HIV testing*
      b. *Consider referral to pediatric infectious disease for more extensive testing*

relationship to ASD as a whole. However, research efforts in this area have not kept pace with developments on the nature, assessment, and treatment of ASD as a whole.

A autistic regression presents with a somewhat different symptom profile than those children who appear delayed from the beginning. Also, a large number of these children have intellectual disability and co-occurring seizure disorders. Additionally, while parents often report that something was amiss with their child prior to autistic regression, no definitive behavioral profile has been established to date that would help better identify those children at risk prior to regression. Much more work is needed to better understand this condition in which apparently developmentally appropriate children demonstrate autistic regression (1).

REFERENCES

1. Matson JL, Kozlowski AM. Autistic regression. *Res Autism Spectr Disord.* 2009;4:340–345.
2. Ritvo ER, Freeman BJ. National society for autistic children definition of the syndrome of autism. *J Pediatr Psychol.* 1977;2:142–145.
3. Scher MS, Kidder BM, Bangert BA. Pediatric epilepsy evaluations from the prenatal perspective. *J Child Neurol.* 2007;22:396–401.
4. Oslejsková H, Dusek L, Makovská Z, Pejcochová J, Autrata R, Slapák I. Complicated relationship between autism with regression and epilepsy. *Neuroendocrinol Lett.* 2008;29:558–570.
5. Ballaban-Gil K, Tuchman B. Epilepsy and epileptiform EEG: association with autism and language disorders. *Ment Retard Dev Disabil Res Rev.* 2000;6:300–308.
6. Malow BA. Sleep disorders, epilepsy, and autism. *Ment Retard Dev Disabil Res Rev.* 2004;10:122–125.

Vegetative Disturbances: Sleep, Eating, and Elimination Problems

SAMPLE CASE

Casey is a 10-year-old young man with autism who is brought to the office by his exhausted parents who continue to struggle with his eating problems. Although Casey has made striking gains in social and language skills, he continues to defy his parents' best efforts at eating anything than highly pureed foods, of which he will only consume chicken, some fruit, and French fries. Exceptional efforts have been made by the family to gradually increase both a variety of type of food and different textures of food, with no success. In addition to concerns to Casey's slight build, the parents spend a great deal of time and money attempting to meet his growing need for nutrition with the volume of pureed foods necessary. Speech evaluation was requested, and a program to reduce oral sensitivity was started. At the same time, additional formal behavioral modification was instituted both at home and at school that focused on classical conditioning. Although some strides were made, after 6 months Casey still resisted most forms of food. Ultimately, he was started on risperidone to help reduce apparent anxiety and compulsivity regarding food choices, as well as other rigidity of thinking. After an additional of 3 months on a combined program of speech and behavioral therapy as well as a low dose of the neuroleptic, Casey ultimately gave up pureed foods and progressed to several different food types and gradually acquired skills to eat simple finger foods without pureeing.

MANAGEMENT OF VEGETATIVE DISTURBANCES

One of the most upsetting issues for some families involves a child whose anxiety or unusual patterns of sleeping, eating, or eliminating are a dominating element of life. Many children with an autistic spectrum disorder (ASD) are observed to have unusual sleep patterns, most often an inability to simply fall asleep, but also not being able to sleep adequately through the night, or to have night terrors. Additionally, many of these children have unusual sensitivities to food and drink, and may present with an exceptionally narrow range of food choices the child will tolerate. Finally, children with an ASD may present with slowness to be toilet trained and in some instances, may manifest phobias or unusual interest in fecal material.

Sleeping Issues

Children with autism are well known to have increased difficulties with sleep, most commonly manifested by delayed onset of sleep, and more disrupted sleep then throughout the night (1–9). History may provide clues to the possibilities of obstructive sleep apnea, gastroesophageal reflux, or seizures, in which case appropriate tests should be requested. When no cause can be found, the use of predictable sleep routines, the absence of televisions or computer screens from the bedroom, as well as behavioral modification are often sufficient (2,5,6). Some research has suggested that errors in melatonin metabolism may be present more often in children with an ASD (10,11). Subsequently, the use of melatonin has been used with some success in children with an ASD diagnosis (3,12). Failing melatonin, the primary care provider (PCP) may consider the use of antihistamines, α_2-agonists, benzodiazepines, chloral hydrate, trazodone, and newer nonbenzodiazepine hypnotic agents (13). Subsequently, for those children and teenagers who may have codiagnoses of epilepsy, aggression, mood disorder, or anxiety, timing the use of those medications at bedtime may be able to resolve sleep issues.

Eating Issues

Although as many as 60% parents of children with an ASD diagnosis report feeding difficulties, parents reported a far smaller number of children with eating disorders, between 5% and 10% (14–16). Research has indicated that children with autism often have a more restricted food range with higher rates of food refusal than their neurotypical peers (16). Additionally, children with ASDs may require specific utensils and food presentation, as well as have tendencies to eat nonedible or other unusual items (14–18).

For children with ASD, the causes of swallowing and feeding disorders are typically complex and multifactorial. The ability to adequately monitor sensory input has been referred to as sensory dysfunction, and can be broadly defined as the inability to adequately monitor incoming sensory information, and may result in a range of responses, including hyperresponsivity, hyporesponsivity, or a mix of the two (19). To complicate matters, children with ASD may be easily overwhelmed by many sensory demands, not the least of which might be a cafeteria or mall, where the sounds of escalating conversations, visual stimuli, odors, and personal space threats may simply force a child to either become aggressive, terrified, withdrawn, or even running from the situation. Finally, rigidity in thinking and requirements for precision of food choices and presentations may make the school cafeteria or a visit to a mall's food court a nightmare for the child.

In order to reduce issues for children, both the behaviors and the environment must be addressed (Table 9.1). As regards behavioral therapy, the parent and therapist will need to work closely to best identify those behaviors that are most troublesome. Enhancing predictability is critical, as is defining specific goals for the therapy. A number of treatment techniques are available, and include sensory-based techniques, such as creating a "sensory diet"; indeed, some

---

TABLE 9.1   Flowchart for Vegetative Disturbance and ASDs

I. *Problems with eating or with eating a limited choice of foods*
   A. *Referral to speech therapy for swallowing study and/or therapeutic approach to oral motor weakness and/or sensory aversion*
   B. *Referral to nutritional consult for tracking caloric intake if weight loss is progressive*
   C. *Referral to behavior therapy for behavior modification to broaden limited diet*
II. *Problems with sleeping*
   A. *Sleep calendar for at least 1 week and ideally 1 month*
   B. *Ensure good sleep hygiene: consistent bedtime, no televisions or electronic screens in bedroom, child has his or her own bed*
   C. *For seriously disturbed sleep in spite of good environmental measures, request sleep study; consider also a routine electroencephalogram*
   D. *For obstructive sleep issues, referral to ENT*
   E. *For nonobstructive sleep issues, consider the use of small dose of α-agonist, such as clonidine, at bedtime to reduce sleep-onset latency*
   F. *For nonobstructive sleep issues, consider the use of small dose of α_2-agonist, such as clonidine, at bedtime to reduce sleep-onset latency*
   G. *For persistence in sleep disorders, consider referral to either pediatric pulmonology, neurology, or sleep specialist*
III. *Problems with elimination*
   A. *Toilet training*
      1. *Delay in toilet training: consider use of behavior management*
      2. *If toilet training is associated with phobias, consider the use of medication to reduce anxiety*
   B. *Inappropriate interest or play with toilet*
      1. *Consider use of behavior management specific to cognitive level*
      2. *Consider use of atypical neuroleptic and/or SSRI to reduce compulsivity*

researchers have described the five essential sensory developments needed for eating: acceptance, touch, smell, taste, and eating (20). In addition to the sensory issues, specific feeding treatment protocols can be very effective in reinforcing the sensory therapies (16). Finally, in rare cases, the PCP may consider the use of medication to reduce anxiety, such as a selective serotonin reuptake inhibitor (SSRI), an atypical neuroleptic, or buspirone.

Toileting Issues

Although toilet training is challenging for many families with small children, it can be particularly frustrating for children with autism, with or without language delays. Most children show signs of emotional and physical readiness as toddlers, typically between 18 months and 3 years of age. In the setting of an autistic spectrum diagnosis, this may not be the case, and is usually determined less by chronological age than developmental readiness. In addition to language and motor delay, children with autism have odd sensory responses oftentimes, even to being soiled. To that end, the following items may be helpful to PCPs in counseling families regarding toilet training a child with autism.

A child who is cognitively ready to attempt toilet training will be able to understand simple commands, being uncomfortable with wearing soiled diapers, and indicating he wishes to be changed. A child with autism may be intellectually able to handle simple commands but actually not perceive any discomfort in wearing soiled diapers. To that end, it may be necessary to place the child in regular underwear and schedule trips to the bathroom every 2 to 3 hours throughout the day so that he becomes cognizant of what it is to have the need to urinate or defecate and associate the use of the bathroom with that need. In addition to autism, some children may also have physical impairments that make using a standard toilet not possible. For these children, working closely with an occupational therapist to customize toileting needs can be very helpful. As for all children, parents need to avoid punishing mistakes or rushing a child to accomplish being toilet trained more quickly than the child is able to proceed.

In older children, social phobias may be present alongside the autism diagnosis, making the use of bathrooms at school problematic. In such cases, a combination of behavior modification, at times with the use of an anxiolytic medication, may be necessary. The same issues can arise at home in the context of painful bowel movements. In such situations, children, regardless of autistic features, may learn to hold making any bowel movements to the point that they acquire constipation and possibly megacolon. Some children, who have exceptionally painful bowel movements, find ways to avoid the toilet altogether, exacerbating the cycle of increasingly hard, painful stools. In such cases, the PCP may need to consider a referral to a pediatric gastroenterologist for the stool softeners and dietary changes, as well as behavior modifications to assist in finding relief for the child. Again, anxiolytics may be of help in this setting.

REFERENCES

1. Cotton SM, Richdale AL. Sleep patterns and behaviour in typically developing children and children with autism, Down syndrome, Prader-Willi syndrome and intellectual disability. *Res Autism Spectr Disord*. 2010;4:490–500.
2. Myers SM. Management of children with autism spectrum disorders. *Pediatrics*. 2007;120(5):1162–1181.
3. Malow BA. Sleep disorders, epilepsy, and autism. *Ment Retard Dev Disabil Res Rev*. 2004;10:122–125.
4. Oyane NM, Bjorvatn B. Sleep disturbances in adolescents and young adults with autism and Asperger syndrome. *Autism*. 2005;9:83–94.
5. Polimeni MA, Richdale AL, Francis AJ. A survey of sleep problems in autism, Asperger's disorder and typically developing children. *J Intellect Disabil Res*. 2005;49:260–268.
6. Wiggs L, Stores G. Sleep patterns and sleep disorders in children with autistic spectrum disorders: insights using parent report and actigraphy. *Dev Med Child Neurol*. 2004;46:372–380.
7. Williams G, Sears LL, Allaed A. Sleep problems in children with autism. *J Sleep Res*. 2004;13:265–268.

8. Patzold LM, Richdale AL, Tonge BJ. An investigation into sleep characteristics of children with autism and Asperger's disorder. *J Paediatr Child Health*. 1998;34:528–533.

9. Schreck KA, Mulick JA, Smith AF. Sleep problems as possible predictors of intensified symptoms of autism. *Res Dev Disabil*. 2004;25:57–66.

10. Tordjman S, Anderson GM, Pichard N, Charbuy H, Touitou Y. Nocturnal excretion of 6-sulpha-toxymelatonin in children and adolescents with autistic disorder. *Biol Psychiatry*. 2005;57:134–138.

11. Kulman G, Lissoni P, Rovelli F, Roselli MG, Brivio, Sequeri P. Evidence of pineal endocrine hypofunction in autistic children. *Neuro Endocrinol Lett*. 2000;21:31–34.

12. Oyane NM, Bjorvatn B. Sleep disturbances in adolescents and young adults with autism and Asperger syndrome. *Autism*. 2005;9:83–94.

13. Owens JA, Babcock D, Blumer J, et al. The use of pharmacotherapy in the treatment of pediatric insomnia in primary care: rational approaches—a consensus meeting summary. *J Clin Sleep Med*. 2005;1: 49–59.

14. Williams, GP, Dalrymple N, Neal J. Eating habits of children with autism. *Pediatr Nursing*. 2000;26: 259–264.

15. Kerwin ME, Eicher PS, Gelsinger J. Parental report of eating problems and gastrointestinal symptoms in children with pervasive developmental disorders. *Child Health Care*. 2005;34:217–223.

16. Twachtman-Reilly J, Amaral SC, Zebrowski PP. Addressing feeding disorders in children on the autism spectrum in school-based settings: physiological and behavioral issues. *Lang Speech Hear Serv Sch*. 2008;39:261–272.

17. Ahearn WH., Castine T, Nault K., Green G. An assessment of food acceptance in children with autism or pervasive developmental disorder-not otherwise specified. *J Autism Dev Disord*. 2001;31:505–511.

18. Schreck KA, Williams K. Food preferences and factors influencing food selectivity for children with autism spectrum disorders. *Res Dev Disabil*. 2006;27:353.

19. Lane SJ, Miller LJ, Hanft BE. Toward a consensus in terminology in sensory integration theory and practice: part 2: sensory integration patterns of function and dysfunction. *Sens Integration Spec Interest Sect*. 2000;23:1–3.

20. Ernsperger L, Stegen-Hanson T. *Just Take a Bite: Easy, Effective Answers to Food Aversions and Eating Challenges*. Arlington, TX: Future Horizons; 2004.

10

Epilepsy and Autistic
Spectrum Disorders

SAMPLE CASE

Joshua is a handsome 5-year-old young man who is brought to the neurodevelopmental disabilities clinic for a neurologic evaluation of his autism. He is currently being well served in the public school where he attends a special communication classroom. Born full term and on time for all milestones until age 18 months, Joshua demonstrates significant loss of language milestones, stereotypes, and social regression. A prior exhaustive genetic and metabolic evaluation has yielded all negative results. Because of his mildly dysmorphic features, his disordered sleep, as well as frequent staring spells, a sleep-deprived electroencephalogram (EEG) is obtained. The EEG yields frequent midparietal spike and slow waves, both in waking and sleeping states, consistent with subclinical seizure activity. The subsequent magnetic resonance imaging (MRI) is unremarkable. One month after starting a broad-spectrum anticonvulsant, parents report a much more verbal and interactive child, although still significantly delayed.

MANAGING EPILEPSY IN AUTISM SPECTRUM DISORDERS

The possibility of an epileptic disorder must be considered in every child with an autistic spectrum disorder (ASD), especially if there is a history of regression. Certainly, many children with an ASD will demonstrate staring spells that is classically a part of the autistic spectrum quite apart from epileptic interference. Further, there is not any apparent evidence that clearly demonstrates causality for epilepsy in those children who present with "typical" ASD. For those children, a screening EEG is no longer considered mandatory, and is the current recommendation for both the American Academy of Pediatrics and the American Academy of Neurology. However, it is important to remember that even subtle epileptic disorders can impair socialization and language development enough that a child can develop an autistic phenotype, and for this reason, keeping the issue of possible clinical and subclinical epilepsy in the differential for the evaluation of a child with an ASD is still important. At the same time, there is certainly no evidence that the routine administration of antiepileptic therapy is either warranted or safe. Those children for whom neither EEGs can either confirm or rule out the presence of an epileptiform disorder must be carefully evaluated and diligently followed over years prior to any commitment to medication. Nevertheless, the relationship between seizure activity and the presence of an ASD is important and complex.

AUTISM AND EPILEPSY: A COMPLEX RELATIONSHIP

Because autism is seen in so many different conditions, it is not at all surprising that children who have autism have a 5% to 40% chance of also having epilepsy (1). What makes the role of the primary care physician even more challenging is that it is difficult to know at what point the two conditions may occur independently of each other or if one has contributed to the evolution of the other. Certainly, well-known epileptic disorders or syndromes are known to present also with autistic phenotypes (2), suggesting that seizure-related activities may actually interfere with the normal neurologic development needed for communication and social skills.

Researchers (3–5) have suggested four mechanisms that best describe the complex relationships between autism and epilepsy:

TABLE 10.1	Epileptic Disorders and Specific Pathologies Potentially Associated with an Epileptic Autistic Regression

Infantile spasms

Early symptomatic partial complex seizures (frontal or temporal)

Acquired epileptic aphasias

Frontal epilepsy with continuous spike waves during slow sleep

Tuberous sclerosis

Hypothalamic hamartoma and epilepsy (4)

1. Both epilepsy and autism may be inherited by independent mechanisms and are not related.
2. Both epilepsy and autism are inherited and develop as the result of the same genetic disorder, such as fragile X, tuberous sclerosis, or even early perinatal insults, such as TORCH infections. Although some researchers believe this is the most common manifestation of both epilepsy and autism, it is important to remember that severe or frequent seizures may contribute to the ongoing cognitive and motor difficulties a child may have (3,6).
3. An epileptic process interferes directly with the function of specific networks involved in the development of human communication and social behavior. Such an example might be the presence of frontal lobe heterotopia that directly interferes with the subsequent neurologic maturation controlling social, linguistic, and motor functions (3,7–10).
4. Children with epileptic syndromes that directly affect the language center may struggle with a wide range of language processes, including but not limited to auditory processing, expressive language, syntactic speech, and pragmatic speech. Although rare, acquired epileptiform aphasias may provide significant clues to a child's delayed onset of language (3,4; Table 10.1). The responsiveness of such conditions to anticonvulsant therapy, however, is highly variable and can be discouraging.

AUTISM AND EPILEPSY: SUGGESTED DIAGNOSTIC AND THERAPEUTIC APPROACH

1. For any child with significant delays, but especially those with rapid regression of previously achieved milestones, in social, motor, or language skills, a screening EEG that includes both waking and sleeping states may be ordered (Table 10.2). Ideally, such a tracing is interpreted by an epileptologist who is well trained in pediatric EEG monitoring.
2. For any child with new-onset seizures in the context of either an ASD or cognitive delay should prompt a screening EEG that includes both waking and sleeping states.
3. If the screening EEG is found to be unremarkable, it is important to ask if a typical event occurred during the tracing. If not, and if concerns persist regarding either regression, new-onset seizures, significant staring spells or odd movements, particularly in the context of a child with either an ASD or cognitive delay, a video and/or overnight EEG may be considered in order to trap a typical event and attempt correlation for any evidence of electric changes.
4. The discovery of abnormal EEG activity may prompt the need for imaging in a child, particularly if focality or lateralizing qualities are seen.
5. Medical management for seizure activities is best initiated by pediatric neurologists, ideally with epilepsy training.
6. Ongoing surveillance will be needed in those children who are placed on anticonvulsant therapies, specifically with routine serologies as dictated by anticonvulsant choice, as well as regular EEG tracings, particularly in the context of any change for the worse in a child who was previously showing progress, as well as in any child who may show adverse responses to medication choices.

TABLE 10.2	Flowchart for Epilepsy and Autistic Spectrum Disorders

I. *ASD and epilepsy*
  A. *Regression or delay of social, motor, language skills*
    1. *Routine EEG: ideally with both sleep and waking tracings*
      a. *If normal EEG, but with no evidence of typical events captured during the tracing, request extended EEG*
        1. *Normal extended EEG*
          i. *Pursue serologic and radiographic evaluation as indicated for regression of milestones*
          ii. *Consider repeating EEG if symptoms persist and are not correlated with existing EEGs*
        2. *Abnormal extended EEG*
          i. *Refer to pediatric neurology*
          ii. *Obtain head imaging, preferably MRI*
          iii. *Genetic evaluation*
          iv. *If anticonvulsants are required, should anticipate a team approach with the pediatric neurologist long term to assist with seizure choice, dosing, and long-term management*
      b. *Abnormal routine EEG*
        1. *Refer to pediatric neurology*
        2. *Obtain head imaging, ideally an MRI*
        3. *Genetic evaluation*
        4. *If anticonvulsants are required, should anticipate a team approach with the pediatric neurologist long term to assist with seizure choice, dosing, and long-term management*

7. Any child who presents with both epilepsy and an ASD must have routine chromosomal analysis and genetic evaluation, as driven by the physical examination. A referral to a genetic clinic is always appropriate in this setting.

REFERENCES

1. Tuchman R, Rapin I. Epilepsy in autism. *Lancet Neurol.* 2002;1:352–358.
2. Besag FM. Behavioral aspects of pediatric epilepsy syndromes. *Epilepsy Behav.* 2004;5(Suppl. 1): S3–S13.
3. Roulet-Perez E, Davidoff V, Prelax AC, et al. Sign language in childhood epileptic aphasia (Landau–Kleffner syndrome). *Dev Med Child Neurol.* 2001;43:739–744.
4. Deonna T, Roulet-Perez E. *Cognitive and Behavioural Disorders of Epileptic Origin in Children. Clinics in Developmental Medicine No. 168.* London: Mac Keith Press; 2005.
5. Roulet-Perez E, Deonna T. Autism, epilepsy, and EEG epileptiform activity. In: Tuchman R, Rapin I, eds. *Autism: A Neurological Disorder of Early Brain Development.* London: Mac Keith Press; 2006:174–188.
6. Lann LA, Renier WO, Aarts WF, et al. Evolution of epilepsy ad EEG findings in Angelman syndrome. *Epilepsia.* 1997;38:195–199.
7. Deonna T, Ziegler AL, Moura-Serra J, Innocenti G. Autistic regression in relation to limbic pathology and epilepsy: report of two cases. *Dev Med Child Neurol.* 1993;35:166–176.
8. Mundy P. The neural basis of social impairments in autism: the role of the dorsal medial-frontal cortex and anterior cingulated system. *J Child Psychol Psychiatry.* 2003;44:793–809.
9. Tuchman R. Autism. *Neurol Clin.* 2003;21:915–932.
10. Allman JM, Watson KK, Tetreault NA, Hakeem AY. Intuition and autism: a possible role for Von Economo neurons. *Trends Cogn Sci.* 2005;9:367–373.

Psychiatric Problems and Autistic Spectrum Disorders

11

SAMPLE CASE

Tony is a 15-year-old young man with a well-established diagnosis of high-functioning autism. He has attended a private special needs school for the last 4 years where he has done quite well. However, without warning, the school shifted policy with regard to suddenly requiring uniforms as well as regimenting the time schedule far more tightly than before. Within a couple of weeks of the new semester when the changes were implemented, the family was alarmed to hear Tony talking repeatedly about his late grandfather instructing him to kill himself and then others. He was very clear about the conversations that he and the grandfather were having. Additionally, Tony began to act more oddly with regard to obsessive behaviors and heightened irritability, with furious outbursts of rage. A referral to a pediatric psychiatric emergency department was made, where the diagnosis of acute psychosis in the context of autism was made. He was started on aripiprazole, removed from the private school, and maintained in a day treatment program until his rage and hallucinations faded. He was ultimately placed in an alternate school setting, with careful and gradual introduction to the classroom and instructors.

MANAGING PSYCHIATRIC ISSUES

By far, most of the psychiatric considerations that arise in the context of autism include obsessive–compulsive disorders with associated anxiety and compulsivities (1–10); attention deficit disorders (11–20); aggression and explosivity (6,21–25); and affective disorders, including depression and bipolar phenotype (9,10,26–34). Rarely, an individual will also present with a comorbid diagnosis of schizophrenia, although not in higher frequency than the nonautistic population (35,36). When questions arise regarding an individual whose autism may have components of self-talk that has always been present, as opposed to a dramatic change in behavior, having an immediate psychiatric assessment can be very helpful.

TABLE 11.1	Flowchart for Evaluation and Management of Psychiatric Issues in ASD

I. *Aggression*
   A. *Determine if threat to self or others; if so, refer to Emergency Department (ED)*
   B. *If not, consider the use of appropriate medication, such as an atypical neuroleptic or anticonvulsant*
II. *Anxiety*
   A. *Determine if threat to self or others; if so, refer to ED*
   B. *If not, consider the use of appropriate medication, such as an atypical neuroleptic or selective serotonin reuptake inhibitor (SSRI)*
III. *Mood disorders*
   A. *Determine if threat to self or others; if so, refer to ED*
   B. *If not, consider the use of a mood stabilizer, such as an atypical neuroleptic or SSRI*
IV. *Psychoses*
   A. *Refer to psychiatric ED*
   B. *Anticipate the need for a psychiatrist for long-term care*

Subsequently, if psychiatric issues arise apart from the core symptoms that have been discussed earlier in this text, it is ideal to seek the assistance of psychiatric professionals to help manage comorbid psychiatric issues that may include bipolar features, depression, or in rare instances, psychoses (Table 11.1).

REFERENCES

1. Rosbrook A, Whittingham K. Autistic traits in the general population: what mediates the link with depressive and anxious symptomatology? *Res Autism Spectr Disord.* 2010;4:415–424.
2. McDougle CJ, Naylor ST, Cohen DJ, Volkmar FR, Heninger GR, Price LH. A double-blind, placebo-controlled study of fluvoxamine in adults with autistic disorder. *Arch Gen Psychiatry.* 1996;53:1001–1008.
3. Sugie Y, Sugie H, Fukuda T, et al. Clinical efficacy of fluvoxamine and functional polymorphism in a serotonin transporter gene on childhood autism. *J Autism Dev Disord.* 2005;35:377–385.
4. Moore ML, Eichner SF, Jones JR. Treating functional impairment of autism with selective serotonin-reuptake inhibitors. *Ann Pharmacother.* 2004;38:1515–1519.
5. Posey DJ, Erickson CA, Stigler KA, McDougle CJ. The use of selective serotonin reuptake inhibitors in autism and related disorders. *J Child Adolesc Psychopharmacol.* 2006;16:181–186.
6. McDougle CJ, Scahill L, Aman MG, et al. Risperidone for the core symptom domains of autism: results from the study by the Autism Network of the Research Units on Pediatric Psychopharmacology. *Am J Psychiatry.* 2005;162:1142–1148.
7. Buchsbaum MS, Hollander E, Haznedar MM, et al. Effect of fluoxetine on regional cerebral metabolism in autistic spectrum disorders: a pilot study. *Int J Neuropsychopharmacol.* 2001;4:119–125.
8. Namerow LB, Thomas P, Bostic JQ, Prince J, Monuteaux MC. Use of citalopram in pervasive developmental disorders. *J Dev Behav Pediatr.* 2003;24:104–108.
9. Owley T, Walton L, Salt J, et al. An open-label trial of escitalopram in pervasive developmental disorders. *J Am Acad Child Adolesc Psychiatry.* 2005;44:343–348.
10. Cheng-Shannon J, McGough JJ, Pataki C, McCracken JT. Second-generation antipsychotic medications in children and adolescents. *J Child Adolesc Psychopharmacol.* 2004;14:372–394.
11. Handen BL, Johnson CR, Lubetsky M. Efficacy of methylphenidate among children with autism and symptoms of attention-deficit hyperactivity disorder. *J Autism Dev Disord.* 2000;30:245–255.
12. Research Units on Pediatric Psychopharmacology Autism Network. Randomized, controlled, crossover trial of methylphenidate in pervasive developmental disorders with hyperactivity. *Arch Gen Psychiatry.* 2005;62:1266–1274.
13. Aman MG. Management of hyperactivity and other acting-out problems in autism spectrum disorder. *Semin Pediatr Neurol.* 2004;11:225–228.
14. Fankhauser MP, Karumanchi VC, German ML, Yates A, Karumanchi SD. A double-blind, placebo-controlled study of the efficacy of transdermal clonidine in autism. *J Clin Psychiatry.* 1992;53:77–82.
15. Jaselskis CA, Cook EH, Fletcher E, Leventhal BL. Clonidine treatment of hyperactive and impulsive children with autistic disorder. *J Clin Psychopharmacol.* 1992;12:322–327.
16. Scahill L, Aman MG, McDougle CJ, et al. A prospective open trial of guanfacine in children with pervasive developmental disorders. Research Units on Pediatric Psychopharmacology (RUPP) Autism Network. *J Child Adolesc Psychopharmacol.* 2006;16:589–598.
17. Posey DJ, Puntney JI, Sasher TM, Kem DL, McDougle CJ. Guanfacine treatment of hyperactivity and inattention in pervasive developmental disorders: a retrospective analysis of 80 cases. *J Child Adolesc Psychopharmacol.* 2004;14:233–241.
18. Jou RJ, Handen BL, Hardan AY. Retrospective assessment of atomoxetine in children and adolescents with pervasive developmental disorders. *J Child Adolesc Psychopharmacol.* 2005;15:325–330.
19. Posey DJ, Wiegand RE, Wilkerson J, Maynard M, Stigler KA, McDougle CJ. Open-label atomoxetine for attention-deficit/hyperactivity disorder symptoms associated with high-functioning pervasive developmental disorders. *J Child Adolesc Psychopharmacol.* 2006;16:599–610.
20. Arnold LE, Aman MG, Cook AM, et al. Atomoxetine for hyperactivity in autism spectrum disorders: placebo-controlled crossover pilot trial. *J Am Acad Child Adolesc Psychiatry.* 2006;45:1196–1205.
21. McCracken JT, McGough J, Shah B, et al. Risperidone in children with autism and serious behavioral problems. *N Engl J Med.* 2002;347:314–321.

22. Arnold LE, Vitiello B, McDougle C, et al. Parent-defined target symptoms respond to risperidone in RUPP autism study: customer approach to clinical trials. *J Am Acad Child Adolesc Psychiatry.* 2003;42: 1443–1450.

23. Vitiello B. An update on publicly funded multisite trials in pediatric psychopharmacology. *Child Adolesc Psychiatr Clin North Am.* 2006;15:1–12.

24. Connor DF, Ozbayrak KR, Benjamin S, Ma Y, Fletcher KE. A pilot study of nadolol for overt aggression in developmentally delayed individuals. *J Am Acad Child Adolesc Psychiatry.* 1997;36:826–834.

25. Ratey JJ, Mikkelsen E, Sorgi P, et al. Autism: the treatment of aggressive behaviors. *J Clin Psychopharmacol.* 1987;7:35–41.

26. Myers SM. Management of children with autism spectrum disorders. *Pediatrics.* 2007;120:1162–1182.

27. Johnson CP, Myers SM; Council on Children with Disabilities. Identification and evaluation of children with autism spectrum disorders. *Pediatrics.* 2007;120:1184–1214.

28. Seltzer MM, Shattuck P, Abbeduto L, Greenberg JS. Trajectory of development in adolescents and adults with autism. *Ment Retard Dev Disabil Res Rev.* 2004;10:234–247.

29. Posey DJ, McDougle CJ. The pharmacotherapy of target symptoms associated with autistic disorder and other pervasive developmental disorders. *Harv Rev Psychiatry.* 2000;8:45–63.

30. Hollander E, Soorya L, Wasserman S, Esposito K, Chaplin W, Anagnostou E. Divalproex sodium vs. placebo in the treatment of repetitive behaviours in autism spectrum disorder. *Int J Neuropsychopharmacol.* 2006;9:209–213.

31. Hollander E, Dolgoff-Kaspar R, Cartwright C, Rawitt R, Novotny S. An open trial of divalproex sodium in autism spectrum disorders. *J Clin Psychiatry.* 2001;62:530–534.

32. Rugino TA, Samsock TC. Levetiracetam in autistic children: an open-label study. *J Dev Behav Pediatr.* 2002;23:225–230.

33. Hardan AY, Jou RJ, Handen BL. A retrospective assessment of topiramate in children and adolescents with pervasive developmental disorders. *J Child Adolesc Psychopharmacol.* 2004;14:426–432.

34. DeLong R. Children with autistic spectrum disorder and a family history of affective disorder. *Dev Med Child Neurol.* 1994;36:674–687.

35. Volkmar FR, Cohen DJ. Co-morbid association of autism and schizophrenia. *Am J Psychiatry.* 1991; 148:1705–1707.

36. Jones N. A meeting of minds. *Nat Med.* 2010;16:353–355.

12 Genetic and Environmental Syndromes Associated with Autistic Spectrum Disorders

SAMPLE CASE

Dustin is a 5-year-old, nonverbal young man who is brought to the office for an initial evaluation of possible autism. His parents note that in addition to never having language, he has a many stereotypical behaviors, including rocking, spinning, and repeated high-pitched squeals when excited. The parents have brought his school records with him, which reveal a full-scale IQ of approximately 55. His physical examination reveals large pinnae, diffusely diminished tone, and velvety skin. He has no other significant finding on either physical or neurologic examination. Routine serologies are normal, as are a routine electroencephalogram (EEG) and cranial magnetic resonance imaging (MRI). The genetic testing, however, reveals an expansion at the *FXMR* gene of greater than 400 repeats, consistent with a diagnosis of fragile X syndrome (FXS). Although Dustin has no siblings, his mother is found to have 120 repeats; his maternal grandfather is found to have 80 repeats. Because of premutation levels, both his mother and his maternal grandfather are referred to their primary care physicians to monitor for associated conditions, specifically premature ovarian failure for his mother, and tremor and ataxia for his grandfather. Subsequently, the child is then referred for speech, occupational, and behavioral modification with subsequent modifications provided in the classroom. No medications were indicated at that time.

GENETIC AND ENVIRONMENTAL CAUSES OF THE AUTISTIC PHENOTYPE

Although the vast majority of children with an autism diagnosis rarely have an etiology identified as the cause for their behavior, there are well-described syndromes that are clearly associated with the development of the autistic behavioral phenotype. For children in whom no clear etiology can be found, the term idiopathic or primary autism is applicable. By contrast, those individuals whose autism is clearly a result of genetic or environmental causes are said to have a secondary autism. At this time, recognizable causes for autism are quite rare, and have been estimated to be not more than 10% and more probably 6% of all cases of secondary autism (1–3). Additionally, the rate of associated cognitive deficit in autism has diminished dramatically from approximately 90% before 1990 to less than 50%, due in large part to the improved psychometric measurement of intellectual capacity in individuals with an autistic spectrum. Subsequently, the comorbid presentation of significantly impaired intellectual capacity in the presence of an autistic spectrum behavior, particularly with associated dysmorphisms on physical examination, is more often consistent with an identifiable disorder (1,4–9). For that reason, it is imperative to be exceptionally attentive to important features of the history and physical that can help identify genetic and environmental causes. It is equally important to avoid a "shotgun" approach and order specifically the genetic or metabolic tests that are indicated by the clinical examination (Table 12.1).

GENETIC SYNDROMES ASSOCIATED WITH AUTISTIC SPECTRUM DISORDERS

Fragile X Syndrome

FXS is regarded as the most common cause of genetically inherited ASD, as well as cognitive delay in males (10,11). The mutations in the fragile X mental retardation 1 gene (*FMR1*), located at Xq23.7, causes a variety of disorders, depending on the length of the cytosine-guanine-guanine

TABLE 12.1	**Flowchart for Evaluation and Management of Genetic and Environmental Syndromes Associated with Autistic Traits**

I. Fragile X
   A. Assess for *FMR1* gene in all children with autism plus cognitive deficiency
   B. *FMR1* carrier state (permutation) in females may be as symptomatic as full expression in males
   C. If an index case is found, genetic counseling must include the extended family
II. Neurocutaneous disorders
   A. Tuberous sclerosis
     1. Two gene products, hamartin and tuberin, can produce the clinical picture
     2. Seizures may present before autistic features
     3. Although TS is an autosomal-dominant condition, most cases are spontaneous mutations. Nevertheless, genetic counseling is warranted if a TS index case is found
   B. Neurofibromatosis type 1
     1. Although less commonly associated with ASD than with LD, NF1 is nevertheless linked
     2. NF1 is autosomal dominant, and if an index case is found, genetic counseling is needed
III. Phenylketonuria
   A. Usually identified in newborn screening
   B. In the context of microcephaly, delay, musty order, and possibility of a missed newborn screen, this should be considered
IV. Angelman syndrome
   A. FISH for 15q deletion syndrome should be requested in cognitively delayed, profoundly impaired language
   B. If clinical picture is strongly suggestive of AS and FISH is negative, request 15q methylation study
V. Rett's syndrome
   A. Classic phenotype is seen in females with autistic regression, microcephaly, seizures, and hand-wringing
   B. Males may present with Rett's syndrome, but presentation is varied; there is increased presentation of Rett's syndrome in males with Klinefelter's syndrome (47XXY)
   C. DNA test for MECP2 is positive in 80% of cases
VI. Smith–Lemli–Opitz syndrome
   A. Rare condition of cholesterol metabolism error
   B. Multiple congenital anomalies, failure to thrive, cognitive delay; occasional poly, syndactyly
VII. Fetal alcohol syndrome
   A. Maternal exposure to alcohol is worse in first trimester, but can yield significant impairment throughout pregnancy
   B. Exposure to alcohol carries a high risk for other substances of abuse
   C. Physical findings may be disproportionately subtle relative to cognitive and emotional issues

(CGG) repetitive sequence. The normal range has 5 to 44 CGG repeats with a mean of 30. Carriers who are usually, but not always, unaffected intellectually have 55 to 200 repeats. However, carriers produce an excessive amount of *FMR1* messenger RNA that can lead to serious illness in later life (12). This includes the fragile X-associated tremor ataxia syndrome in approximately 40% of men and 8% of women (12–14).

The full mutation is associated with greater than 200 CGG repeats. Physical features for FXS include long face; prominent and long ear pinnae; high-arched palate; mitral valve prolapsed; dilated aortic arch; flat feet; hyperextensible finger joints in childhood; macroorchidism (testicle volume greater than 30 ml bilaterally in adulthood); soft or velvet-like skin (15,16). The full mutation occurs in 1 in 2,500 alleles, and the permutation occurs in 1 per 130 to 250 females and in 1 per 250 to 810 males (17). Therefore, genetic testing should be carried out in all children and adults with autism, ASDs and intellectual disability of unknown etiology (16,18–20). Once an individual is identified with an *FMR1* mutation, a careful family history will often reveal many other family members who are either carriers or significantly affected by FXS. Genetic testing and counseling are therefore recommended for the extended family. Being vigilant when an individual presents with an autistic behavioral phenotype to the possibility of a comorbid diagnosis of fragile X is important, because up to 50% of individuals with genetically confirmed fragile X demonstrate some autistic traits (8).

Neurocutaneous Syndromes

Two conditions are most commonly associated with the appearance of an autistic behavior. The first, tuberous sclerosis (TS) (1,21–25) is characterized by hypopigmented macules, fibroangiomas, kidney lesions, central nervous system hamartomas, seizures, cognitive deficiency, and autistic behaviors. TS is a dominantly inherited disorder, with two gene locations at 9q and 16p. However, most cases are new mutations, and the absence of positive family history should not be a deterrent to examining a child with a Wood's lamp to examine for possible hypopigmented lesions.

Although less commonly associated with ASDs, neurofibromatosis type 1 (NF1) can also present with cognitive impairment as well as autistic features. NF1 is characterized by café-aulait macules and freckling in the axillary and inguinal regions, neurofibromas, and ocular Lisch nodules, and although autosomal dominant, it is most often associated with new mutations at 17q (26). NF1 is more commonly associated with learning disabilities rather than autism.

Phenylketonuria

Fortunately, phenylketonuria is rare in the United States because of newborn screening, and subsequently, it is rarely associated with cognitive deficit and ASDs (27). However, in children in whom there is a reason to suspect missed standard newborn screenings, screening for phenylketonuria would be an important consideration, particularly in the context of cognitive delays, microcephaly, seizures, a musty smell, and autistic features. Early detection permits dietary modification that can markedly improve a child's clinical outcome.

Angelman Syndrome

Angelman syndrome (AS) (28–31) is a particularly severe disorder in which the individual does not have the maternally expressed gene, called the ubiquitin-protein ligase gene (*UBE3A*) on 15q through deletion, paternal uniparental disomy, or imprinting errors. Such individuals are typically very delayed, often completely nonverbal, and hypotonic initially as children, with a subsequent development of ataxia and spasticity. Individuals with AS also typically have seizures, which can often be refractory to standard medication. Screening for a deletion of 15q can be accomplished by commercial fluorescence in situ hybridization (FISH) testing; however, a negative FISH result in a child who clinically fits an AS diagnosis should also have a methylation study to assess for uniparental disomy.

Rett's Syndrome

A rare disorder, genetic testing for Rett's syndrome (RS) (32–38) should be considered in all girls who present with a regressive autistic phenotype, and particularly in girls who demonstrate microcephaly, seizures, and hand-wringing compulsions. DNA testing at the *MECP2* gene is confirmatory in 80% of cases. Although possible to manifest in boys, it is far less common and presents with greater variability.

Smith–Lemli–Opitz Syndrome

Also quite rare, Smith–Lemli–Opitz syndrome (SLOS) (39) is an autosomal-recessive disorder that is caused by errors in cholesterol metabolism, and has a prevalence of not more than 1 in 20,000 children, most often of Caucasian or Scandinavian descent. Children with SLOS have microcephaly, syndactyly of second and third toes, and occasional polydactyly, with malformations often seen in the heart, kidney, gastrointestinal tract, genitalia, with hypotonia. Because recurrence occurs at 25% within families, it is an important consideration in this clinical context.

ENVIRONMENTAL DISORDERS

Fetal Alcohol Syndrome

Children who are exposed to alcohol during gestation have an increased risk for ASDs, as well as other behavioral and cognitive problems. Careful history may yield important information for a possible diagnosis of fetal alcohol syndrome (FAS), and can provide significant help for a child in his or her academic years, because it is associated more often with not just ASDs, but mood disorders, learning disabilities, and Attention Deficit Hyperactivity Disorder (ADHD) (40,41). Physical features include a smooth philtrum, small palpebral fissures, and thin upper vermillion. Central nervous system complaints include poor memory, cognition, judgment, and executive function, often with poor self-regulation, hyperactivity, and attention problems. Other organs may also be included, which include cardiac, renal, ocular, and dental problems.

Multisubstance Abuse Syndrome

Although there are fewer controlled studies looking specifically at the role of illegal substances as a direct causation of ASDs, certainly evidence exists for the increased prevalence of cognitive, emotional, and motor delays in infants whose mothers have exposed them in utero to cocaine, heroin, and other street drugs.

Second-Hit Theory

Regardless of the mechanism, a review of studies published in the past 50 years revealed convincing evidence that most cases of ASDs result from interacting genetic factors. However, the expression of the autism gene(s) may be influenced by environmental factors. Although still theory only, these factors may in fact represent a "second-hit" event that primarily occurs during fetal brain development. That is, environmental factors may modulate already existing genetic factors responsible for the manifestation of ASDs in individual children.

SUMMARY

Although known genetic and environmental causes for ASDs are still rare, investigation for clinically driven studies is important. The presence of cognitive impairment as well as dysmorphic features in the context of a child with an ASD should always prompt genetic investigation, as well as a thorough history for possible maternal exposure to infection, drugs, or alcohol. When a genetic cause is identified, genetic counseling not only for the parents but for the extended family as well may be critically important.

REFERENCES

1. Johnson CP, Myers SM; Council on Children with Disabilities. Identification and evaluation of children with autism spectrum disorders. *Pediatrics.* 2007;120:1183–1215.
2. Chakrabarti S, Fombonne E. Pervasive developmental disorders in preschool children. *JAMA.* 2001; 285:3093–3099.
3. Chakrabarti S, Fombonne E. Pervasive developmental disorders in preschool children: confirmation of high prevalence. *Am J Psychiatry.* 2005;162:1133–1141.
4. Autism and Developmental Disabilities Monitoring Network Surveillance Year 2000 Principal Investigators; Centers for Disease Control and Prevention. Prevalence of autism spectrum disorders: Autism and Developmental Disabilities Monitoring Network, Six Sites, United States, 2000. *MMWR Surveill Summ.* 2007;56(1):1–11.
5. Autism and Developmental Disabilities Monitoring Network Surveillance Year 2002 Principal Investigators; Centers for Disease Control and Prevention. Prevalence of autism spectrum disorders: Autism

and Developmental Disabilities Monitoring Network, 14 Sites, United States, 2002. *MMWR Surveill Summ.* 2007;56(1):12–28.

6. Yeargin-Allsopp M, Rice C, Karapurkar T, Doernberg N, Boyle C, Murphy C. Prevalence of autism in a US metropolitan area. *JAMA.* 2003;289:49–55.

7. Wiggins LD, Baio J, Rice C. Examination of the time between first evaluation and first autism spectrum diagnosis in a population-based sample. *J Dev Behav Pediatr.* 2006;27:S79–S87.

8. Demark JL, Feldman MA, Holden JJ. Behavioral relationship between autism and fragile X syndrome. *Am J Ment Retard.* 2003;108:314–326.

9. Honda H, Shimizu Y, Rutter M. No effect of MMR withdrawal on the incidence of autism: a total population study. *J Child Psychol Psychiatry.* 2005;46:572–579.

10. Hagerman PJ, Hagerman RJ. The fragile X premutation: a maturing perspective. *Am J Hum Genet.* 2004;74:805–816. [Published correction appears in *Am J Hum Genet.* 2004;75:352.]

11. Rogers SJ, Wehner DE, Hagerman R. The behavioral phenotype in fragile X: symptoms of autism in very young children with fragile X syndrome, idiopathic autism, and other developmental disorders. *J Dev Behav Pediatr.* 2001;22:409–417.

12. Hagerman RJ. Fragile X syndrome and associated disorders in adulthood. *Continuum Lifelong Learning Neurol.* 2009;15(6):32–49.

13. Coffey SM, Cook K, Tartaglia N, et al. Expanded clinical phenotype of women with the FMR1 premutation. *AM J Med Genet A.* 2008;52(pt 6):1009–1016.

14. Jacquemont S, Hagerman RJ, Leehey MA, et al. Penetrance of the fragile X-associated tremor/ataxia syndrome in a permutation carrier population. *JAMA.* 2004;291(4):460–469.

15. Hagerman RJ, Berry-Kravis E, Kaufmann WE, et al. Advances in the treatment of fragile X syndrome. *Pediatrics.* 2009;123(1):378–390.

16. Hagerman PJ, Hagerman RJ. The fragile X premutation: a maturing perspective. *Am J Hum Genet.* 2004;74:805–816. [Published correction appears in *Am J Hum Genet.* 2004;75:352.]

17. Hagerman RJ, Hall DA, Coffey S, et al. Treatment of fragile X-associated tremor ataxia syndrome (FXTAS) and related neurological problems. *Clin Interv Aging.* 2008;3(2):251–262.

18. Rogers SJ, Wehner DE, Hagerman R. The behavioral phenotype in fragile X: symptoms of autism in very young children with fragile X syndrome, idiopathic autism, and other developmental disorders. *J Dev Behav Pediatr.* 2001;22:409–417.

19. Watson MS, Leckman JF, Annex B, et al. Fragile X in a survey of 75 autistic males. *N Engl J Med.* 1984;310:1462.

20. Hagerman RJ. Physical and behavioral phenotype. In: Hagerman FJ, Hagerman PJ, eds. *Fragile X: Diagnosis, Treatment and Research.* 3rd ed. Baltimore, MD: Johns Hopkins University Press; 2002:3–109.

21. Smalley SL. Autism and tuberous sclerosis. *J Autism Dev Disord.* 1998;28:407–414.

22. Baker P, Piven J, Sato Y. Autism and tuberous sclerosis complex: prevalence and clinical features. *J Autism Dev Disord.* 1998;28:279–285.

23. Wiznitzer M. Autism and tuberous sclerosis. *J Child Neurol.* 2004;19:675–679.

24. Curatolo P, Porfirio M, Manzi B, Seri S. Autism in tuberous sclerosis. *Eur J Paediatr Neurol.* 2004; 8:327–332.

25. Curatolo P. Tuberous sclerosis: genes, brain, and behavior. *Dev Med Child Neurol.* 2006;48:404.

26. Lauritsen M, Ewald H. The genetics of autism. *Acta Psychiatr Scand.* 2001;103:411–427.

27. Baieli S, Pavone L, Meli C, Fiumara A, Coleman M. Autism and phenylketonuria. *J Autism Dev Disord.* 2003;33:201–204.

28. Clayton-Smith J, Laan L. Angelman syndrome: a review of the clinical and genetic aspects. *J Med Genet.* 2003;40:87–95.

29. Thatcher KN, Peddada S, Yasui DH, LaSalle JM. Homologous pairing of 15q11–13 imprinted domains in brain is developmentally regulated but deficient in Rett and autism samples. *Hum Mol Genet.* 2005;14:785–797.

30. Lopez-Rangel E, Lewis ME. Do other methyl-binding proteins play a role in autism? *Clin Genet.* 2006;69:25.

31. Niemitz EL, Feinberg AP. Epigenetics and assisted reproductive technology: a call for investigation. *Am J Hum Genet.* 2004;74:599–609.

32. Ham AL, Kumar A, Deeter R, Schanen NC. Does genotype predict phenotype in Rett syndrome? *J Child Neurol.* 2005;20:768–778.

33. Kerr AM, Ravine D. Review article: breaking new ground with Rett syndrome. *J Intellect Disabil Res.* 2003;47:580–587.

34. Kerr AM, Prescott RJ. Predictive value of the early clinical signs in Rett disorder. *Brain Dev.* 2005;27(Suppl. 1):S20–S24.

35. Kerr A. Annotation: Rett syndrome—recent progress and implications for research and clinical practice. *J Child Psychol Psychiatry.* 2002;43:277–287.

36. Einspieler C, Kerr AM, Prechtl HF. Abnormal general movements in girls with Rett disorder: the first four months of life. *Brain Dev.* 2005;27(Suppl. 1):S8–S13.

37. Ravn K, Nielsen JB, Uldall P, Hansen FJ, Schwartz M. No correlation between phenotype and genotype in boys with a truncating *MECP2* mutation. *J Med Genet.* 2003;40:e5.

38. Moog U, Smeets EE, van Roozendaal KE, et al. Neurodevelopmental disorders in males related to the gene causing Rett syndrome in females (*MECP2*). *Eur J Paediatr Neurol.* 2003;7:5–12.

39. Elias E, Giampietro P. Autism may be caused by Smith-Lemli-Opitz syndrome (SLOS). Presented at Annual Clinical Genetics Meeting; March 17–20, 2005; Dallas, TX.

40. Aronson M, Hagberg B, Gillberg C. Attention deficits and autistic spectrum problems in children exposed to alcohol during gestation: a follow-up study. *Dev Med Child Neurol.* 1997;39:583–587.

41. Clarren, S.K. (2005). A thirty year journey from tragedy to hope. Foreword to in: Buxton B, ed. *Damaged Angels: An Adoptive Mother Discovers the Tragic Toll of Alcohol in Pregnancy iv–xiv*. New York: Carroll & Graf.

13 Individuals with Exceptional Gifts and Autistic Spectrum Disorders: Autistic Savants

SAMPLE CASE

Bill, at age 47, had been living in a group home environment all of his adult life and had been reasonably successful at maintaining a nonskilled job at a local grocery store, as well as at home, where his routine had been carefully established and rarely disrupted. He had an unusual gift for being able to name on which day of the week any particular day would fall, even many years into the future. It was a phenomenal gift and one that he enjoyed a great deal. However, he still required careful structuring in his day. Without it, he would become very agitated and would remove himself from his routine duties and pleasures. Bill qualified for the diagnosis of an autistic savant; however, he was unable to live independently.

EXCEPTIONAL SKILLS WITH EXCEPTIONAL IMPAIRMENTS: FINDING WAYS TO ENHANCE THE WHOLE

Literature suggests that the prevalence of savant abilities in autism may be as high as 10%, compared to less than 1% in individuals without a diagnosis of autism (1). However, the truly exceptional savant's who is capable of performing rapid difficult mathematical problems; calculate calendar dates years in the past or future; demonstrate exceptional memory for obscure details; or exhibit exceptional musical or artistic abilities, is in fact quite rare, at least in the clinical setting. Although many individuals with autistic spectrum disorders (ASD) may be exceptionally bright with astonishing gifts in language, art, or music, a distinction is often made between autistic savants and prodigious savants, with prodigious savants numbering less than 100 worldwide. In contrast to an autistic savant, Treffert and others have suggested that a prodigious savant is an individual whose talent would render him or her a prodigy regardless of whether the individual also has an ASD. Studies have suggested that male-to-female ratio approaches 6:1, with an estimate of 50% of all savants as having autism and the other 50% with a wide range of learning disabilities and cognitive disorders (2,3).

Those individuals who are considered autistic savants, regardless of whether their talent is truly prodigious, are typically described as having exceptional talent in the realm of memory, calculations, especially for dates and the rapid calculation of seemingly complex numbers such as all prime numbers, as well as music, art, and language (4–8). Difficulties arise when the presence of an ASD in addition to the savantism renders day-to-day living overwhelming for the individual.

Research suggests that during early development, people with autism can "overdevelop" a normal brain circuit and develop prodigious capacity, despite their severe cognitive and behavioral handicaps. Brain mapping has suggested that autistic savant development might be associated with a developmental disorganization of the neural circuits, facilitating the emergence of these particular networks (9). Intellectual testing between savant and nonsavant individuals has shown statistical difference in digit span; however, the significance of this is uncertain (10).

SUMMARY

The presence of exceptional talent in the context of an individual with an ASD can yield exceptional challenges. Having an environment that does not risk exploitation of the individual is critically important (Table 13.1). Additionally, the recognition that an individual is allowed a creative

TABLE 13.1	Flowchart for Assisting Individuals with Autistic Savant Syndrome

I. *Splintered exceptional skills in the context of significant social ± communication impairments*
  A. *Avoid exploitative settings*
  B. *Behavior modification can maximize gifts and at the same time address communicative impairments*
II. *Most commonly expressed in mathematics, memory, musical, or artistic skills*

outlet for his or her talent in the context of a safe day-to-day environment is also a critically important plan for the individual. As psychometric testing has become far more sensitive to individuals with an ASD relative to their cognitive strengths and weaknesses, creating the best learning and living environment can be tailor-made to the individual in a way that was not always possible in prior decades. Working with exceptionally gifted people can be very rewarding, but also challenging; when it is also in the context of an ASD, even more creativity and patience may be needed to find best ways to support the individual.

REFERENCES

1. Treffert DA. The savant syndrome: an extraordinary condition. A synopsis: past, present, future. *Philos Trans R Soc Lond B Biol Sci*. 2009;364:1351–1357.
2. Howlin P, Goode S, Hutton J, Rutter M. Savant skills in autism: psychometric approaches and parental reports. *Philos Trans R Soc Lond B Biol Sci*. 2009;364:1359–1367.
3. Mottron L, Belleville S, Stip E. Proper name hypermnesia in an autistic subject. *Brain Lang*. 1995; 53(3):326–350.
4. Pring L, Hermelin B, Heavey L. Savants, segments, art and autism. *J Child Psychol Psychiatry*. 1995; 36(6):1065–1076.
5. Anderson M, O'Connor N, Hermelin B. A specific calculating ability. *Intelligence*. 1998;26:383–403.
6. Heaton P, Wallace GL. Annotation: the savant syndrome. *J Child Psychol Psychiatry*. 2004;45: 899–911.
7. Snyder A, Mitchell D. Is integer arithmetic fundamental to mental processing? The mind's secret arithmetic. *Proc R Soc Lond B Biol Sci*. 1995;(266):587–592.
8. Pring L. Savant talent. *Dev Med Child Neurol*. 2005;47:500–503.
9. Boddaert N, Barthelemy C, Poline JB, Samson Y, Brunelle F, Zibovicius M. Autism: functional brain mapping of exceptional calendar capacity. *Br J Psychiatry*. 2005;187(1):83–86.
10. Bolte S, Poustka F. Comparing the intelligence profiles of savant and nonsavant individuals with autistic disorder. *Intelligence*. 2004;32:121–131.

14 Adults Living with an Autistic Spectrum Diagnosis

SAMPLE CASE

A family requested consultation with a physician to discuss concerns regarding Matthew's transition from high school to adult years. An hour was blocked for what was anticipated as a lengthy and detailed discussion. Matthew, a handsome, quiet 19-year-old young man had received exceptionally good services for his high-functioning autistic spectrum disorder (ASD) throughout his elementary, junior, and senior high years. Regardless, he still exhibited significant gaze avoidance, with a monotone speech that was concrete in content. Additionally, he clearly had limited understanding, interest, or judgment about money, dating, or living independently.

The clinician, parents, and Matthew participated in a kind but frank discussion that included a review of his interests, as well as his and his parents' ideas about the future conversation about what he was most interested in doing and how his parents envisioned their future with him. He had become proficient at computer programming and preferred this to all other activities. Although he was not interested in dating, he did enjoy participating in a very accepting and warm church program. When he had been in high school, he struggled with social isolation and some depression about "being different". Although that was less of an issue currently, it was suggested that as he started his college classes, perhaps visiting with a known and trusted counselor of those years might be helpful to help with adapting to a college campus. Further, his capacity for distraction was such that the parents judged that a driver's license was not appropriate anytime soon. The college semester work-load was discussed, and included Matthew using a combination of both computer-based distance learning and on-campus classes. Finally, the total work load was discussed, and Matthew was very open to limiting the total amount of course work to not more than 9 hours a semester, at least to start. Finally, the parents were advised to seek the guidance of a family law specialist to provide legal protection for him in the case that they might pre-decease him. Matthew and both his parents were in agreement that if his parents were not available, he would be safer if his living arrangements involved assistance from either a family member or family friend.

ADULTS WITH AN ASD

Like so much of the literature in ASD, all individuals with an ASD are so very unique that no cookbook approach will work. However, reviewing specific needs for all adults with or without an ASD can yield a custom fit in what otherwise is an "off the rack" world. Core symptoms,

TABLE 14.1	Suggested Areas for Review in Anticipatory Care

1. *Work environment:* unskilled, skilled, professional work options
2. *Financial management:* access to cash, savings, and retirement funds
3. *Home environment:* family of origin; group home, semiautonomous, independent
4. *Transportation:* provided transport by group or family home; mass transit; driving
5. *Socialization:* access to socialization guided by interests and best mental health practices
6. *Medical needs:* understanding of how aware an individual is to his or her own medical needs
7. *Emotional needs:* behavior modification; group therapy; cognitive therapy as needed
8. *Legal needs:* legal protection for funding and living arrangements in the absence of family

TABLE 14.2	Flowchart for Adults with ASD

a. *As patients, these individuals typically require extra time scheduled in an appointment to review with compulsive care issues regarding health care decisions*

b. *The PCP may wish to involve a psychologist to help the individual explore best ways to maintain a balance between social withdrawal and social interaction*

c. *Legal guidance is needed especially in situations where an adult with an ASD may need intermittent, regular part-time or full-time assistance of other adults*

d. *Avoid "warehousing"; independent living may not be optimal for socially vulnerable individuals, despite normal or near-normal cognition*

e. *Individuals who have very mild ASD and very high functioning may need only cognitive counseling as issues with dating, career, marriage, and children arise*

including socialization, anxiety, and odd behaviors, often diminish over decades, but in the context of unexpected routines or poorly supported environments, they can certainly reappear (1). A checklist that can be used would include reviewing issues relative to work, home, career, and legal protection (2; Table 14.1). Concerns should be initiated by family and guided as appropriate by the primary care physician (PCP; Table 14.2).

REFERENCES

1. Davis TE, Hess JA, Moree BN, et al. Anxiety symptoms across the lifespan in people diagnosed with autistic disorder. *Res Autism Spectr Disord*. 2010;40:266–267.
2. Grandin T, Duffy K. *Developing Talents: Careers for Individuals with Asperger's Syndrome and High Functioning Autism*. Shawnee Mission KS: AAPC; 2008.

15 Ethical Considerations in the Primary Medical Care of Individuals with an Autistic Spectrum Disorder

SAMPLE CASE

A family brought their 12-year-old autistic daughter with them to the office, and had scheduled a prolonged visit to discuss how to best approach her approaching menses and their very valid fear that she would "freak out" when that started, because she had struggled with toileting to great degrees. Indeed, she still had difficulty consistently cleaning herself after elimination of both urine and feces. Additionally, the parents stated that although they were able to provide for her safety for most of her day, they were very worried about her vulnerability as she got older to unwanted sexual demands. Tasha, who was present, spent most of the hour quietly rocking throughout the examination. Her verbal skills were limited to simple phrases with poor eye contact. She had been maintained on several medications to reduce aggression and assist in sleep.

The hour was spent reviewing a number of options. What the family felt would not be acceptable was for the young woman to become pregnant, now or in the future, given her lack of comprehension of her own personal issues or capacity to care for an infant. It was ultimately determined by the family that she had become much better in the last year about personal hygiene, with far less emotional upset than she had experienced as a child. Further, it was suggested that because she had matured a great deal, that perhaps starting with monthly hormonal injections to make her menses more predictable and somewhat lighter would be a reasonable first step. The parents agreed that they would prefer to avoid any surgical sterilization at this time and agreed to see a local obstetrician/gynecologist who had particular expertise in working with young women with cognitive impairments. Two years later, Tasha has started her periods and had done very well at personal care and hygiene. She seemed to not mind the monthly injections, and the family is pleased with their decision. They understand that although the monthly injections will prevent pregnancy, it will not prevent sexually transmitted illness. Long-term goals for the family include allowing her to stay in a family home, if possible, their own. Further, the family has found an attorney with expertise and interest in family law, particularly in the context of caring for an impaired minor child, and has subsequently established legal protection that states which family members would assume her care if her parents should predecease her.

ETHICAL CONCERNS IN ASD

Because the presentation of ASD is highly variable, with a range of severity as well as types of impairment, the application of ethical principles requires as sensitive an application. Clinical ethics have been described as "the identification of morally correct actions and the resolution of ethical dilemmas in medical decision making through the application of moral concepts and rule to medical situations" [1]. One of the best utilized system of bioethics was developed by Beauchamp and Childress, and is based on four essential ethical principles, specifically, respect for autonomy, nonmaleficence, beneficence, and justice (Table 15.1). In the context of caring for the primary medical needs of individuals with an ASD, this system is quite useful [2].

TABLE 15.1	Flowchart for Ethical Concerns for Individuals with Autistic Traits

I. *Autonomy when possible*
  A. *Avoid warehousing whenever possible*
  B. *Important to respect the individual's need for privacy and still provide protection as needed, especially in areas of finance, relationships, sexuality, and bearing children*
  C. *Having a "safe place" to talk to a trusted counselor or mentor can be life-saving*
  D. *Long-term goals may or may not include independent living, even for individuals with seemingly "mild" impairment*

II. *Beneficence*
  A. *Maintain vigilance to neglect of health because of a seeming "oblivious" sense of need*
  B. *Actively working in the community to find best support systems for individuals with ASD is proactive and yields significant rewards for the PCP practice as well as individual*

III. *Nonmaleficence*
  A. *Approach to sexuality should begin with education and when the individual is cognitively ready*
  B. *Reproduction rights should be measured by each individual, and in the "never competent" individual, a standard of best interest should be used, such that a cognitively impaired person who cannot provide self-care does not become pregnant*

IV. *Justice*
  A. *The active involvement of individuals with an ASD in a primary care practice helps provide needed care for a significant portion of the population who would not otherwise receive it*

V. *Dignity always*

CONCEPT FOR RESPECT FOR AUTONOMY AND ASD

Regardless of the degree of impairment from an ASD, all individuals seek autonomy to at least some degree. However, individuals who have limited speech, understanding, or capacity for judgment may need less autonomy than an approach of least infringement on those areas which are most important to the individual's sense of personhood. Subsequently, wherever autonomy can be respected without risking undue medical, physical, or emotional harm, the primary care provider (PCP) is urged to consider ways in which the individual can best be served.

CONCEPT OF BENEFICENCE AND ASD

Beneficence is the moral duty to promote good. In the context of working with individuals with an ASD, beneficence would imply the active attempt to rescue an imperiled patient if and only if the patient is at risk to suffer significant loss or damage; the physician's action is needed, singly or in concert with others, to prevent or minimize the loss; the physician is capable, alone or with others, of attempting the necessary action; there is a high probability that individual or group action will be successful; enacting physician will not incur significant risks, costs, or burdens; and the patient's expected benefits outweigh the possible harms, costs, or burdens that the physician could incur (3).

In the context of an individual with an ASD, the physician may be required to encourage medical assessments when the individual in his or her oblivion to personal issues would otherwise be unconcerned. Such an approach could possibly incur against the earlier principle of autonomy. However, such concerns must be balanced against being aware to what degree an individual patient is in fact truly cognizant of inherent medical danger. One example might be the 42-year-old highly functioning woman with autism whose mammogram revealed an early cancerous lesion. Rather than realize the risks she was taking was inherently dangerous, she essentially took a year to find a single surgeon who would do a very limited lumpectomy when in fact more rigorous surgery by that point was needed. It is unclear had the woman understood the real risks for some speed, that her surgery might have happened sooner and she might have avoided death 5 years later. Documenting that a patient truly understands the consequences of any medical concern is best done by having the patient or his or her guardian repeat back in their own words their understanding of medical risks. In individuals with an ASD, such discussions may take much longer than in individuals who have less difficulty with socialization or communication skills (4,5).

THE CONCEPT OF NONMALEFICENCE AND ASD

The ethical duty of nonmaleficence is steeped in oldest medical tradition of *primum non nocere*, or "above all, do no harm" (1,2). Perhaps where this is most applicable in the care of individuals with ASD is seen frequently in the context of reproductive rights of individuals with ASD. In low-functioning individuals with severe cognitive deficits and communication, for whom caring for an infant would be impossible, arriving at ways to protect the individual against fertility as well as sexually transmitted illness requires a thoughtful and careful approach. For those individuals who are higher functioning with mild ASDs, early education at puberty that is direct but nonthreatening is important. Ultimately, the decision for long-term relationships, sexual encounters, and marriage must be guided by the ongoing sensitivity to the individual's capacity for self-care and care for others. Nonmaleficence is then needed for the careful protection of the individual against unwanted pregnancy or sexually transmitted illness, but weighed against the need and capacity for autonomy (6–9).

THE CONCEPT OF JUSTICE AND ASD

In the context of clinical medicine, the concept of justice is often used to refer to society's system for the distribution of resources on the basis of concepts of fairness and desert, including distributions of services on the basis of individual need, individual effort, societal contribution, merit or desert, and personal contribution (1,6). In the context of caring for individuals with an ASD, the involvement of PCPs for the needs of the ASD community is critically important. The current availability for specialists who work in autism is very scarce; as of 2010, there are not more than 700 specialists in total for neurodevelopmental disabilities, and behavioral developmental pediatricians nationwide (7,8). However, using the Center for Disease estimates at 1 in 110 individuals with an ASD (9), the United States faces a significant shortfall of 700,000 children younger than 18 years with a probably ASD (4). Clearly, the role of PCP becomes critically important as we as a medical community attempt to meet the challenge of serving the individual with an ASD.

PREDICTING LONG-RANGE NEEDS: HOW A MULTIDISCIPLINARY APPROACH HELPS

Because living with an ASD affects so many stages of life, it is very helpful for the PCP to establish a network of specialists within the community. For instance, for pediatricians, the use of education liaisons; occupational, speech, and behavioral therapists; and medical subspecialists as needed is usually essential for a holistic approach to a child's needs in the ASD context. Alternatively, for primary care specialists who work with individuals across the life span, having access to life skills counselors; educators with special expertise in specialty colleges, educational programs, and state-related support programs for severely impaired individuals; social workers to help facilitate community resources for group homes or transportation issues, can all be very helpful. It typically requires that the PCP actively network with the community leaders in autism. And as with all patients, as an individual moves from childhood to adolescence to adulthood and on to senior years, the issues of ASD will often modify relative to biological and emotional needs.

REFERENCES

1. Bernat JL. Mental retardation. In: *Ethical Issues in Neurology*. 3rd ed. Philadelphia, PA: Lippincott Williams & Wilkins; 2008:386–407.

2. Beauchamp TL, Childress JF. *Principles of Biomedical Ethics*. 5th ed. New York: Oxford University Press, 2001.

3. Pelligrino ED, Thomasma DC. *For the Patient's Good: The Restoration of Beneficence in Health Care*. New York: Oxford University Press; 1988:25–36.

4. Dayan J, Minnes P. Ethical issues related to the use of facilitated communication techniques with persons with autism. *Can Psychol*. 1995;36:183–189.

5. American Board of Pediatrics. Workforce and research: number of diplomat certificates granted through December 2009. Retrieved August 7, 2010, from https://www.abp.org/ABPWebStatic/#murl%3D%2FABPWebStatic%2FaboutPed.html%26surl%3D%2Fabpwebsite%2Fstats%2Fnumdips.htm.

6. Nichols S, Blakeley-Smith A. "I'm not sure we're ready for this ..." Working with families toward facilitating healthy sexuality for individuals with autism spectrum disorders. *Soc Work Ment Health*. 2010; 8:72–91.

7. Kalyva E. Teachers' perspectives of the sexuality of children with autism spectrum disorders. *Res Autism Spectr Disord*. 2010;4:433–437.

8. Glasberg B. Review of "Making sense of sex: A forthright guide to puberty, sex, and relationships for people with Asperger's syndrome." *J Autism Dev Disord*. 2010;40:392–393.

9. Lotan G, Ells C. Adults with intellectual and developmental disabilities and participation in decision making: ethical considerations for professional-client practice. *Intellect Dev Disabil*. 2010;48:112–125.

Section Three:

Therapeutic Approaches

Environmental Approaches

16

IMPORTANCE OF ENVIRONMENT AS A THERAPEUTIC COMPONENT

Home, school, and work environments are critically important for therapies, tutoring, and medication.

Predictability and consistent routine in twenty-first-century American life are increasingly rare and difficult components. However, for any person with a diagnosis under the autistic spectrum, it is the commitment to routine by family, caregivers, educators, and indeed the autistic individual him- or herself that is most consistently predictive of success over the long term (1,2).

HOME: THE STARTING POINT FOR CONSISTENCY IN BEHAVIOR AND LANGUAGE

The economic reality for most young families in this country means both parents work; that a child's home has a 27% chance of being headed by a single parent. The prevalence of blended families tends to be underreported, but of those families that experience divorce, possibly as many as 75% will enter into a blended family and remarriage (1–4). Finding ways to incorporate behavior and language habilitation for a child can be challenging in not only carving time out for multiple therapeutic sessions a week, but also finding ways for all caregivers to provide consistency in the critically important techniques suggested by therapists.

After the diagnosis of an autism spectrum disorder has been made by testing, it is optimal to have all caregivers participate in conference-based office visits to ensure not only that all parties are involved in the decision making of therapies and medications, but that consistency for eating, sleeping, and toilet training is practiced in all settings in which the child may call home.

In the case of divorce, particularly those fraught with conflict, it is highly recommended that the caregivers participate with professional family counseling in order to maximize communication on behalf of the child with autism whose progress will be completely dependent on the adults in his or her life to make consistency a priority.

EDUCATIONAL TOOLS CAN BE IMPORTED TO THE HOME ENVIRONMENT AS WELL

Section IV details at length issues regarding American public school services and procedures. However, in the context of environment as an important concern for the therapeutic milieu, mention is made here also of comprehensive programs for young children as well as older children and teenagers.

Data repeatedly and conclusively show that the earlier a child is enrolled into intensive intervention, the better is the long-term outcome (5–7). A high degree of structure is uniformly implemented among all the various programs, as well as the inclusion of a family member. Such intensive therapies are recommended by many of these programs to have active involvement of the child, a minimum of 25 hours a week, 12 months a year, with systematically planned goals for communication, socialization, and cognitive tasks (8–11).

Home and classroom environments are able to employ a range of strategies, depending on what is most appropriate to the child. Applied behavior analysis (ABA) has, in recent years, moved from an inconceivable expense for most families to one that is still quite expensive, but now more often available in slightly different programming. ABA methods are used to increase and maintain desirable adaptive behaviors, reduce interfering maladaptive behaviors or narrow the conditions under which they occur, teach new skills, and generalize behaviors to new environments or situations (12–14). ABA has been shown to be highly effective over the last 50 years, and continues to be an important mainstay of autism rehabilitation. Children who receive early intensive behavioral treatment such as ABA show substantial and long-lasting improvements in communication, intellect, socialization, and adaptive behaviors (12–19).

Structured teaching is a model for environmental support that emphasizes structure as its core component. One such method, Treatment and Education of Autistic and Communication related handicapped Children (TEACCH) (20,21) has particular emphasis on the visual, timely, and physical structure of the child's environment. Components of TEACCH and of any structured teaching program for children with autism include predictable sequence of events, visual schedules, routines with flexibility, structured work/activity systems, and visually structured activities—all centered on the careful organization of the environment (20–26).

More recently, pediatricians have been urged to adopt a broader approach not only for screening for functionality, but for implementing broader approaches to intervention that are based more broadly on play and reciprocal interactions (27). Early evidence exists that play-based or social-pragmatic interventions that address the core deficits in autism including the capacity to engage with others, humor, problem solving, and emotional thinking have been overlooked in the need to provide rigid structure in earlier versions of environmental support (27–31).

In the final analysis, any individual carrying a diagnosis under the autistic spectrum must have careful and tailored approaches to his or her environment, including school, home, and when possible, work. Evidence continues to reinforce that the earlier and more inclusive the intervention, the more successful individuals are. Environment must take into consideration not just consistency in schedules and physical space, but also functionally grounded relationship intervention in which play and affection are centered.

WORK AND PLAY

Freud famously said that love and work are the cornerstones of our humanity. This applies even to children whose "job" it is to achieve the highest level of functioning that a child's neurologic system will permit, including finding ways to be relational as possible. The earliest possible and intensive use of therapies that emphasize environmental consistency with relational and functional goals continues to be the first element to crafting a careful program of therapeutics for any individual with an autistic disorder.

REFERENCES

1. Maher M. (2010). U.S. children in single-mother families, PRB.org. Retrieved May 31, 2010, from http://www.prb.org/pdf10/single-motherfamilies.pdf
2. U.S. Department of Health and Human Services, Administration for Children and Families, Office of Planning, Research, and Evaluation, VII. Formation and maintenance of two-parent families. Sixth Annual Report to Congress (2004). Retrieved May 31, 2010, from www.acf.hhs.gov/programs/ofa/data-reports/annualreport6/chapter07/chap07.htm
3. Halpern-Meekin S. Heterogeneity in two-parent families and child well-being. In: Conference Papers—American Sociological Association, 2006 Annual Meeting, Montreal, 1–44.
4. Myers SM. Management of children with autism spectrum disorders. *Pediatrics*. 2007;120:1162–1182.
5. Shevell MI. Present conceptualization of early childhood neurodevelopmental disabilities. *J Child Neurol*. 2009;25:120–125.
6. Johnson CP, Myers SM; and the Council on Children with Disabilities. Identification and evaluation of children with autism spectrum disorders. *Pediatrics*. 2007;120(5):1183–1205.
7. Lord, C., McGee, JP, eds. *National Research Council, Committee on Educational Interventions for Children with Autism. Educating Children with Autism*. Washington, DC: National Academies Press; 2001.

8. Olley JG. Curriculum and classroom structure. In: Volkmar FR, Paul R, Klin A, Cohen D, eds. *Handbook of Autism and Pervasive Development Disorders*. 3rd ed. Vol II. Hoboken, NJ: John Wiley & Sons; 2005:863–881.

9. Dawson G, Osterling J. Early intervention in autism. In: Guralnick MJ, ed. *The Effectiveness of Early Intervention: Second Generation Research*. Baltimore, MD: Brookes; 1997:307–326.

10. Harris SL, Handelman JS, Jennett HK. Models of education intervention for students with autism: home, center, and school-based programming. In: Volkmar FR, Paul R, Klin A, Cohen D, eds. *Handbook of Autism and Pervasive Developmental Disorders*. 3rd ed. Vol II. Hoboken, NJ: John Wiley & Sons; 2005:10443–1054.

11. Bregman JD, Zager D, Gerdtz J. Behavioral interventions. In: Volkmar FR, Paul R, Klin A, Cohen D, eds. *Handbook of Autism and Pervasive Developmental Disorders*. 3rd ed. Vol II. Hoboken, NJ: John Wiley & Sons; 2005:897–924.

12. Lorimer PA, Simpson RL, Myles BS, et al. The use of social stories as a preventative behavioral intervention in a home setting with a child with autism. *J Posit Behav Interv.* 2002;453–460.

13. Taylor BA. Teaching peer social skills to children with autism. In: Maurice C, Green G, Foxx RM, eds. *Making a Difference: Behavioral Intervention for Autism*. Austin, TX: Pro-Ed; 2001:83–96.

14. Weiss MJ, Harris SL. Teaching social skills to people with autism. *Behav Modif.* 2001;25:785–802.

15. Campbell JM. Efficacy of behavioral interventions for reducing problem behavior in persons with autism: a quantitative synthesis of single-subject research. *Res Dev Disabil.* 2003;24:120–138.

16. Heflin LJ. Increasing treatment fidelity by matching interventions to contextual variables within the educational setting. *Focus Autism Other Dev Disabil.* 2001;16:93–101.

17. Van Bourgondien ME, Reichle NC, Campbell DG, Mesibov GB. The Environmental Rating Scale (ERS): a measure of the quality of the residential *environment* for adults with *autism. Res Dev Disabil.* 1998;19(5):381–394.

18. Gray C. The impact of home and school interventions on the adjustment of children with *autism* spectrum disorders. *Dissertation Abstracts International: Section B: The Sciences and Engineering.* 2010; 70(8-B):5161.

19. Mesibov GB, Shea V, Schopler E. *The TEACCH Approach to Autism Spectrum Disorders*. New York: Kluwer Academic/Plenum; 2005.

20. Lord C, Schopler E. The role of age at assessment, developmental level, and test in the stability of intelligence scores in young autistic children. *J Autism Dev Disord.* 1989;19:483–499.

21. Marcus LM, Lansing M, Andrews CE, Schopler E. Improvement of teaching effectiveness in parents of autistic children. *J Am Acad Child Psychiatry.* 1978;17:625–639.

22. Mesibov GB. Formal and informal measures on the effectiveness or the TEACCH programme. *Autism.* 1997;1:25–35.

23. Schopler E, Mesibov GB, Baker A. Evaluation of treatment for autistic children and their parents. *J Am Acad Child Psychiatry.* 1982;21:262–267.

24. Short AB. Short-term treatment outcome using parents as co-therapists for their own autistic children. *J Child Psychol Psychiatry.* 1984;25:443–458.

25. Venter AC, Lord C, Schopler E. A follow-up study of high functioning autistic children. *J Child Psychol Psychiatry.* 1992;33:489–507.

26. Greenspan SI, Brazelton TB, Cordero J, et al. Commentary: guidelines for early identification, screening, and clinical management of children with autism spectrum disorders. *Pediatrics.* 2008;121(4): 828–830.

27. Greenspan SI, Wieder S. An integrated developmental approach to interventions for young children with severe difficulties in relating and communicating. *Zero to Three.* 1997;15(5):5–18.

28. Greenspan SI, Wieder S. A functional developmental approach to autism spectrum disorders. *J Assoc Pers Sev Handicaps.* 1999;24(3):147–161.

29. Wieder S, Greenspan S. Can children with autism master the core deficits and become empathetic, creative, and reflective? A ten to fifteen year follow-up of a subgroup of children with autism spectrum disorders (ASD) who received a comprehensive developmental, individual-difference, relationship-based (DIR) approach. *J Dev Learn Disord.* 2005;9:1–29.

30. Greenspan SI, Wieder S. *Engaging Autism: The Floortime Approach to Helping Children Relate, Communicate, and Think*. Reading, MA: Perseus Books; 2005.

31. Solomon R, Necheles J, Ferch C, Ruckman D. Pilot study of a parent training program for young children with autism. *Autism.* 2007;11(3):205–224.

17 Nonpharmacologic Therapeutic Options

In addition to environmental supports and structure, the addition of formal therapies has been shown to be critically important for many children and teenagers. Although speech and occupational therapies are particularly important for early onset of intervention, the introduction of appropriate therapies at any point in development, from childhood to the adult years, can yield significant improvement in an individual's independence and capacity for interaction with others.

Of these, there are at least four major domains where the primary care physician may wish to prescribe regular therapeutic sessions. These include speech therapy, occupational therapy, social skills therapy, and most recently, a subset of social and communication skills therapy—virtual reality-based therapy. In our practice, a common approach is to have a child with an autistic spectrum disorder (ASD) diagnosis to participate in speech and occupational therapy on a minimum of twice-weekly sessions for each modality. As the child's speech improves, and per the recommendation of the speech therapist, the child may also be enrolled in formal social skills coaching. All recommendations must be tailored to the child's diagnosis, needs, and the accessibility of therapists. It is possible to "overtherapize" a child, and for that reason, care must be taken to ensure that the child has blocks of unstructured time to relax and participate in those activities he or she finds most entertaining.

SPEECH AND LANGUAGE THERAPY

A variety of approaches have been used and found to be very helpful for enhancing communication in individuals with ASDs. These include methodologies such as didactic and naturalistic behavioral therapy (Discrete Trial Teaching (DTT), Applied Behavioral Analysis (ABA), verbal behavior, natural language paradigm, pivotal response training, and milieu teaching) have all been studied. Additional support exists for a developmental pragmatic model as well, and it includes programs such as social communication emotional regulation transactional support (SCERTS), Denver model, Relationship Development Intervention (RDI), and the Hanen model (1–4).

Most individuals can dramatically improve their social speech, regardless of age, prerequisite strengths or weaknesses, and intellectual capacity. What has been shown to be ineffective has been the traditional low-intensity, pull-out service delivery models seen commonly in public school settings. Speech therapists are most successful in their work when they have the opportunity to work closely with care givers, teachers, and support personnel in order to promote functional communication in natural settings throughout the day.

Augmentative and alternative communication modalities, such as American sign language, picture and communication boards, and even the child's best gestural commands—all can be effective in building communication skills (1,2,5,6). The picture exchange communication system is one popularly used communication system that is used in many children and teenagers with a wide variety of neurodevelopmental disorders.

The primary care physician is encouraged to seek out what resources are available in his or her community. Any prescription provided for speech therapy must include the diagnosis of an ASD in order for the speech therapist to design the best possible program and goals.

OCCUPATIONAL THERAPY

Perhaps more than many of the suggested therapeutics in this short chapter, the role of occupational therapy for individuals with ASDs has gendered significant controversy over the last

20 years. Certainly, there are programs that have arisen that have yielded reduced anxiety and improved cognitive functioning, as well as therapies that are not helpful or have not yet been shown to provide significant relief. However, across the board, there are increasing numbers or well-done, peer-reviewed, double-blinded studies to help identify those therapies that have the most yield from those that have no yield and are potentially financially ruinous. Among those, sensory integration has been recently identified as being particularly salient to the occupational therapeutic support of individuals with ASDs as well as relationship-based, interactive interventions (7–9).

However, the entire "field" of sensory integration is so broad as to warrant a cautionary tone; while some techniques may have value, many do not. Standardization is still needed for many of the techniques utilized, including but not limited to issues of wearing weighted vests, skin brushing, joint compression, and others. What has not been borne out have been offshoots of sensory integration, most specifically cranial sacral therapy, which has no peer-reviewed, double-blinded research in which to base its use and is discouraged by this author.

Primary care providers are encouraged to have families seek evaluations with board-certified occupational therapists, who are able to provide clear goals and techniques prior to the onset of therapy.

SOCIAL SKILLS THERAPY

A relatively new concept in the form of therapeutic milieu, the idea of how to make and maintain friendships has often been included in private school and some public school settings for many generations, in the context of "friends" groups. However, when children present with significant impairment to processing nuanced social clues because of innate problems in processing environment, using a social skills therapist can be instrumental to providing critically important skills that a child can use the rest of his or her life.

Some limited research has been done, but much more is needed (10). Children who appear to benefit most from social skills training are those whose family is also involved in implementing techniques at home and through the week. Practicing "scripted" dialogue in a social setting with peers can be invaluable to elevate awareness for children who often seem oblivious to social cues. Practiced eye contact with appropriate dialogues in a variety of settings can be the difference between being able to stay in a mainstream classroom to being removed to one with potentially fewer options socially and academically.

Insurance rarely reimburses for social skills training, making the often exorbitant cost for private social skills coaching cost often the most commonly cited reason for families not participating. However, even brief exposures of 6 to 8 weeks can be incredibly helpful for those children who are truly at sea about how to start interactions with peers. Families are encouraged to seek out those programs in their community that specifically coach social skills to children and teenagers with pragmatic and syntactic language problems.

VIRTUAL REALITY THERAPEUTICS

Perhaps one of the most exciting developments in the last decade has been the emergence of very sophisticated computer-based software, which enables individuals with social and communication impairment to use avatars in which to interact with other individuals in safe, supervised, and counseling-based environments. Although expensive, immersive virtual reality (VR) has the potential to be very helpful in coaching socialization and self-confidence. Some studies have observed an increase in both gaze duration and vocalizations (11). Researchers have also found that VR is particularly helpful for people with ASDs because of its structure, opportunity for repetition, affective engagement, and the ability for the individual to control his or her own environment (12). VR offers its exclusive advantage of making it possible to explicitly show imaginary or magic transformations of how an object can act as if it were a different one, which is useful for training in both abstract concepts and imagination understanding.

Again, this is a new field that needs more extensive investigation to best understand which programs are best for the therapeutic endeavor. Additionally, unsupervised participation on Internet sites can be exceptionally risky for individuals with ASDs, and for that reason, the discussion of VR is limited to strict applications of therapy-driven and supervised work.

REFERENCES

1. National Research Council, Committee on Educational Interventions for Children with Autism. In: Lord C, McGee JP, eds. *Educating Children with Autism*. Washington, DC: National Academies Press; 2001.
2. Goldstein H. Communication intervention for children with autism: a review of treatment efficacy. *J Autism Dev Disord*. 2002;32:373–396.
3. Paul R, Sutherland D. Enhancing early language in children with autism spectrum disorders. In: Volkmar FR, Paul R, Klin A, Cohen D, eds. *Handbook of Autism and Pervasive Developmental Disorders*. 3rd ed. Vol II. Hoboken, NJ: John Wiley & Sons; 2005:946–976.
4. Myers S, Johnson CP & American Academy of Pediatrics Council on Children with Disabilities. Management of children with autism spectrum disorders. *Pediatrics*. 2007;120(5):1162–1182.
5. American Speech-Language-Hearing Association, Ad Hoc Committee on Autism Spectrum Disorders. Principles for speech-language pathologists in diagnosis, assessment, and treatment of autism spectrum disorders across the life span; 2005. Retrieved June 4, 2010, from http://www.asha.org/public/speech/disorders/Autism.htm.
6. DeThorn LS, Johnson CJ, Walder L, Mahurin-Smith J. When "Simon Says" doesn't work: alternatives to imitation for facilitating early speech development. *Am J Speech Lang Pathol*. 2009;18(2):133–145.
7. Petrus C, Adamson, SR, Block L, Einarson SJ, Sharifenjad M, Harris SR. Effects of exercise interventions on stereotypic behaviours in children with autism spectrum disorder. *Physiother Can*. 2008;60(2):134–145.
8. Arbesman M, Lieberman D. Evidence-based practice resources: autism spectrum disorders. *OT Pract*. 2009;14(22):25–27.
9. Wauang Y, Wang C, Huang M, Su C. The effectiveness of simulated developmental horse-riding. *Adapt Phys Activ Q*. 2010;27(2):113–126.
10. Epp KM. Outcome-based evaluation of a social skills program using art therapy and group therapy for children on the autism spectrum. *Child Sch*. 2008;30(1):27–36.
11. Herrera G, Jordaon R, Vera L. Abstract concept and imagination teaching through virtual reality in people with autism spectrum disorders. *Technol Disabil*. 2006;18(4):173–180.
12. Mineo BA, Ziegler W, Gill S, Salkin D. Engagement with electronic screen media among students with autism spectrum disorders. *J Autism Dev Disord*. 2009;39(1):172–187.

Pharmaceutical Approaches 18

This chapter seeks to provide basic information for psychopharmacology with regard to drug choice, dosing suggestions, and basic approaches to use these agents for individuals with autistic spectrum disorder (ASDs). However, for more extensive reading on psychopharmacology, the reader is encouraged to review the following excellent texts:

- *The Prescriber's Guide (Essential Psychopharmacology Series) (Paperback)*, Stephen Stahl, 3rd ed., Cambridge Press, 660 pp.
- *Stahl's Essential Psychopharmacology: Neuroscientific Basis and Practical Applications* (Essential Psychopharmacology Series), 3rd ed., Cambridge Press, 1132 pp.
- *Kaplan and Sadock's Synopsis of Psychiatry: Behavioral Sciences/Clinical Psychiatry, North American Edition*, 10th ed., Lippincott Williams & Wilkins, 1472 pp.
- For a truly extensive and review of psychiatric medications and conditions, both adult and pediatric, *Kaplan and Sadock's Comprehensive Textbook of Psychiatry* (2-volume set, 4884 pp.; Lippincott Williams & Wilkins) is in its 9th ed. and provides an in-depth reading on current psychiatric practices.

As the third leg of management for ASDs, pharmaceutical intervention is typically the last step after the implementation of environmental and therapeutic milieus have been implemented. The role of medication should serve as a supplement to other therapeutic options, and with the shared understanding among family and practitioner, there is no easy fix. Medications can be life saving, quite literally, for a family in crisis and besieged by the tyranny of an aggressive, nonverbal child. Indeed, recent surveys indicate that nearly half of children and adolescents (1–3) and up to three-quarters of adults with ASDs are treated with psychotropic medication. Older age, lower adaptive skills and social competence, and higher levels of challenging behavior are associated with the likelihood of medication use (3). The evidence regarding the efficacy of psychopharmacologic interventions in patients with ASDs has been detailed in recent reviews (4–7). However, medication is never to be used in the absence of appropriate emotional and environmental supports.

Incorporating the routine use of psychopharmaceuticals into any practice, whether primary or specialized, requires thorough training and facility with these complex agents. It is important to also scheduling protected time within the practitioner's day to sit with families and review and update goals for academics, psychosocial concerns, and real and potential problems with medication choices. Finally, it is important for the family to realize that it takes months to years, rather than days to weeks, to achieve optimal dosing of medication. For that reason, it is imperative for families to be especially vigilant in participating in environmental and nonmedication-based therapeutics.

When treating children for symptoms related to autism, several rules must apply first and foremost. These are as follows:

1. The use of psychoactive medication is invariably best utilized when counseling is an integral part of the treatment plan.
2. Stimulants often aggravate the anxiety typically seen in individuals with ASD and must be used with caution.
3. Medications used for aggression, such as the neuroleptics, may be administered at night and can often help with comorbid sleep disturbances.
4. When possible, start low and go slow.

5. Avoid changing dosing on more than one medication at a time, and unless an adverse event should occur, permit 1 to 2 weeks minimum before increasing the dose.

6. Should an adverse event occur, monitor withdrawal of any psychoactive drug with care and follow strict pharmacologic guidelines relative to its withdrawal to prevent an exacerbation of the adverse event as well as to prevent any specific withdrawal syndromes, such as in selective serotonin reuptake inhibitors (SSRIs).

7. Careful documentation regarding even mildly adverse responses to medication is instrumental in guiding further decision making.

8. Before any medications are prescribed, careful goal setting by the family, including the patient with autism if appropriate, as guided by the practitioner, is critical. Medication choices are symptom driven, with careful prioritizing of type and severity of symptoms.

9. Maintaining a behavior calendar on the part of the caregivers as well as educators can be critically important to understanding how successful or unsuccessful any particular medication, as well as adjusted doses, has been.

10. After medication is initiated, ongoing and regular visits that are protected 30- to 60-minute visits are necessary for optimal titration and management.

Psychopharmacology may be considered for maladaptive behaviors such as aggression, self-injurious behavior, repetitive behaviors, such as perseveration, obsessions, compulsions and stereotypic movements, sleep disturbance, mood liability, irritability, anxiety, hyperactivity, inattention, destructive behavior, or other disruptive behaviors (1,3,8). After treatable medical causes and modifiable environmental factors have been ruled out, a therapeutic trial of medication may be considered in behavioral symptoms which may be causing significant impairment in functioning and are suboptimally responsive to behavioral interventions.

Also, it is important to remember that children with ASDs have the same basic health care needs as children without disabilities and benefit from the same health-promotion and disease-prevention activities, including immunizations (1). In addition, they may have unique health care needs that relate to the underlying etiologic conditions, such as epilepsy, neurocutaneous disorders, or prenatal injuries. As in all children, a holistic approach to prioritizing medical and behavioral concerns will drive medication choices and dosing.

SAMPLE CASE: JOSHUA

Joshua came to our clinic when he was 9 year old and whose diagnosis of high-functioning autism was missed for many years. Since age 5 years, he had been managed with a range of both short- and long-acting stimulants for what was believed to be severe Attention Deficit Hyperactivity Disorder (ADHD) combined, with significant impulsivity. Additionally, Joshua demonstrated encyclopedic knowledge of lawn mowers, weed eaters, and lawn trimmers. Although this was worrisome, it was not at first associated as being necessarily autistic given his high verbal skills. However, the methylphenidate and Dexedrine products had had only minimal success and in fact, seemed to increase agitation, although his focus was minimally improved for a short time. After extensive psychometric assessment, it was determined that he in fact was more appropriately diagnosed as having high-functioning autism. The stimulants were discontinued, and the family and child were placed into a combination of therapies, including 20 hours a week of applied behavioral analysis (ABA).

The child was also placed in private speech therapy (ST) with particular emphasis on pragmatic and syntactic speech. After approximately 6 months of speech therapy, the child was then "graduated" to social skills coaching with a group of three other boys his same age. He also received occupational therapy (OT) once to twice a week to reduce sensory defensiveness. Additional OT goals included both fine motor training to reduce his illegible handwriting and work on a computer to facilitate keyboard skills.

During this time, Joshua was placed on a low dose of risperidone at 0.25 mg in the AM and then ultimately BID. Over the next 6 months he was ultimately titrated to risperidone at 0.5 mg BID.

TABLE 18.1	Selected Potential Medications Options for Targeted Symptoms	

Target Symptom Cluster	Potential Coexisting Diagnoses	Selected Medication Considerations
Repetitive behavior, behavioral rigidity, obsessive–compulsive symptoms	Obsessive–compulsive disorder, stereotypic movement disorder	SSRIs (fluoxetine, fluvoxamine, citalopram, escitalopram, paroxetine, sertraline) (5–10) Atypical antipsychotic agents (risperidone, aripiprazole, olanzapine, quetiapine, ziprasidone) (11–18) Valproic acid (19,20)
Hyperactivity, impulsivity, inattention	Attention-deficit hyperactivity disorder	Stimulants (methylphenidate, dextroamphetamine, mixed amphetamine salts) (21–24) α_2-Agonists (clonidine, guanfacine) (25–32) Atomoxetine (33–35) Atypical antipsychotic agents (risperidone, aripiprazole, olanzapine, quetiapine, ziprasidone) (11–15,17,18)
Aggression, explosive outbursts, self-injury	Intermittent explosive disorder	Atypical antipsychotic agents (risperidone, aripiprazole, olanzapine, quetiapine, ziprasidone) α_2-Agonists (clonidine, guanfacine) (11–15,17,18) Anticonvulsant mood stabilizers (levetiracetam, topiramate, valproic acid) (19,20,36,37) SSRIs (fluoxetine, fluvoxamine, citalopram, escitalopram, paroxetine, sertraline) (5–10) β-Blockers (propranolol, nadolol, metoprolol, pindolol) (38)
Sleep dysfunction	Circadian rhythm sleep disorder, dyssomnia—not otherwise specified	Melatonin (39,40) Ramelteon (41) Antihistamines (diphenhydramine, hydroxyzine) (29,42) α_2-Agonists (clonidine, guanfacine) (28,30,31,42) Mirtazapine (32)
Anxiety	Generalized anxiety disorder, anxiety disorder—not otherwise specified	SSRIs (fluoxetine, fluvoxamine, citalopram, escitalopram, paroxetine, sertraline) (5–10) Buspirone (43) Mirtazapine (32)

(continued)

TABLE 18.1	Selected Potential Medications Options for Targeted Symptoms *(continued)*	
Target Symptom Cluster	Potential Coexisting Diagnoses	Selected Medication Considerations
Depressive phenotype (marked change from baseline, including symptoms such as social withdrawal, irritability, sadness or crying spells, decreased energy, anorexia, weight loss, sleep dysfunction)	Major depressive disorder, depressive disorder—not otherwise specified	SSRIs (fluoxetine, fluvoxamine, citalopram, escitalopram, paroxetine, sertraline) (5–10) Mirtazapine (32)
Bipolar phenotype (behavioral cycling with rages and euphoria, decreased need for sleep, manic-like hyperactivity, irritability, aggression, self-injury, sexual behaviors)	Bipolar I disorder, bipolar disorder—not otherwise specified	Anticonvulsant mood stabilizers (carbamazepine, gabapentin, lamotrigine, oxcarbazepine, topiramate, valproic acid) (1–4,39,44–46) Atypical antipsychotic agents (risperidone, aripiprazole, olanzapine, quetiapine, ziprasidone) (11–18,32,44)

Summaries: 1–4,39,45,46.

Although he had marked improvement in social skills and reduction in anxiety, he was still quite poorly focused. At that time, a small dose of an extended methylphenidate salt was added, Concerta 18 mg. Over the ensuing months, it was gradually increased to Concerta 36 mg in the AM.

Now as an adult, Joshua is maintained on risperidone 0.5 mg BID and no stimulant medication. He lives in his family's home in a separate living area. He describes himself as happy, and his family would agree. He maintains a very successful lawn business, and although not able to drive more than a few blocks at a time without significant anxiety, he does quite well in this setting. The profits he makes from his lawn company are placed into both a savings and checking account, and the impulsivity to buy many lawn mowers and weed eaters is checked with careful structure in his environment. The family has existing legal safeguards in place to protect Joshua if they should predecease him.

SAMPLE CASE: BRIAN

Brian was referred to our clinic at age 4 years for evaluation of rage events and global delay. After careful history and physical examination, it was determined that he had bilaterally enlarged gastrocnemius muscles, and a subsequent serum creatine kinase CK level was found to be in excess of 12,000 IU. His Duchenne's muscular dystrophy (DMD) was confirmed, and he was referred to a pediatric neuromuscular clinic for assistance in managing his muscle disease. At the same time, psychometric testing revealed pervasive developmental delay—not otherwise specified (PDD-NOS). His rages were made initially worse with prednisone as prescribed by the neuromuscular team; however, a small dose of risperidone was added with limited success. During this time, the family and child participated in play therapy as well as speech therapy for his autistic symptoms. He was also followed closely by both occupational and physical therapy. Over the next 12 months, Brian was gradually increased on his risperidone, which helped his moods but caused significant weight gain. He was then changed to Abilify 2.5 mg and was able to stabilize his weight gain but continued to have much more stable moods with reduced anxiety and aggression.

Two years later, Brian is still ambulatory and verbal to complex sentences, with significantly improved reciprocity in conversation. He is currently stabilized on Abilify at 2.5 mg daily.

PHARMACEUTICAL MANAGEMENT OF AUTISTIC TRAITS

Because all medication approaches are currently centered only on the palliative care, rather than preventative or curative aspects of autism, any choice of medication must be weighed judiciously for its risk-to-benefit ratio for potential side effects, cost, and any risk of withdrawal. Nevertheless, the judicious use of medication in combination with environmental changes and therapeutic interventions can truly make a dramatic improvement in the life of an individual whose autistic traits pose significant impairments. Table 18.1 is provided merely as a reference point for selection of medications for symptoms; the practitioner is encouraged to seek additional information as needed from the manufacturer's instructions and appropriate pharmaceutical guides.

REFERENCES

1. Myers SM. Management of children with autism spectrum disorders. *Pediatrics.* 2007;120:1162–1182.
2. Johnson CP, Myers, SM; Council on Children with Disabilities. Identification and evaluation of children with autism spectrum disorders. *Pediatrics.* 2007;120:1184–1214.
3. Seltzer MM, Shattuck P, Abbeduto L, Greenberg JS. Trajectory of development in adolescents and adults with autism. *Ment Retard Dev Disabil Res Rev.* 2004;10:234–247.
4. Posey DJ, McDougle CJ. The pharmacotherapy of target symptoms associated with autistic disorder and other pervasive developmental disorders. *Harv Rev Psychiatry.* 2000;8:45–63.
5. Hollander E, Phillips A, Chaplin W, et al. A placebo controlled crossover trial of liquid fluoxetine on repetitive behaviors in childhood and adolescent autism. *Neuropsychopharmacology.* 2005;30:582–589.
6. McDougle CJ, Naylor ST, Cohen DJ, Volkmar FR, Heninger GR, Price LH. A double-blind, placebo-controlled study of fluvoxamine in adults with autistic disorder. *Arch Gen Psychiatry.* 1996;53:1001–1008.
7. Moore ML, Eichner SF, Jones JR. Treating functional impairment of autism with selective serotonin-reuptake inhibitors. *Ann Pharmacother.* 2004;38:1515–1519.
8. Posey DJ, Erickson CA, Stigler KA, McDougle CJ. The use of selective serotonin reuptake inhibitors in autism and related disorders. *J Child Adolesc Psychopharmacol.* 2006;16:181–186.
9. Buchsbaum MS, Hollander E, Haznedar MM, et al. Effect of fluoxetine on regional cerebral metabolism in autistic spectrum disorders: a pilot study. *Int J Neuropsychopharmacol.* 2001;4:119–125.
10. Namerow LB, Thomas P, Bostic JQ, Prince J, Monuteaux MC. Use of citalopram in pervasive developmental disorders. *J Dev Behav Pediatr.* 2003;24:104–108.
11. McCracken JT, McGough J, Shah B, et al. Risperidone in children with autism and serious behavioral problems. *N Engl J Med.* 2002;347:314–321.
12. Arnold LE, Vitiello B, McDougle C, et al. Parent-defined target symptoms respond to risperidone in RUPP autism study: customer approach to clinical trials. *J Am Acad Child Adolesc Psychiatry.* 2003;42:1443–1450.
13. McDougle CJ, Scahill L, Aman MG, et al. Risperidone for the core symptom domains of autism: results from the study by the Autism Network of the Research Units on Pediatric Psychopharmacology. *Am J Psychiatry.* 2005;162:1142–1148.
14. Shea S, Turgay A, Carroll A, et al. Risperidone in the treatment of disruptive behavioral symptoms in children with autistic and other pervasive developmental disorders. *Pediatrics.* 2004;114(5);1447–1448.
15. Research Units on Pediatric Psychopharmacology Autism Network. Risperidone treatment of autistic disorder: longer-term benefits and blinded discontinuation after 6 months. *Am J Psychiatry.* 2005;162:1361–1369.
16. Troost PW, Lahuis BE, Steenuis MP, et al. Long-term effects of risperidone in children with autism spectrum disorders: a placebo discontinuation study. *J Am Acad Child Adolesc Psychiatry.* 2005;44:1137–1144.
17. Cheng-Shannon J, McGough JJ, Pataki C, McCracken JT. Second-generation antipsychotic medications in children and adolescents. *J Child Adolesc Psychopharmacol.* 2004;14:372–394.

18. DeLong R. Children with autistic spectrum disorder and a family history of affective disorder. *Dev Med Child Neurol.* 1994;36:674–687.

19. Hollander E, Soorya L, Wasserman S, Esposito K, Chaplin W, Anagnostou E. Divalproex sodium vs. placebo in the treatment of repetitive behaviours in autism spectrum disorder. *Int J Neuropsychopharmacol.* 2006;9:209–213.

20. Hollander E, Dolgoff-Kaspar R, Cartwright C, Rawitt R, Novotny S. An open trial of divalproex sodium in autism spectrum disorders. *J Clin Psychiatry.* 2001;62:530–534.

21. Quintana H, Birmaher B, Stedge D, et al. Use of methylphenidate in the treatment of children with autistic disorder. *J Autism Dev Disord.* 1995;25:283–294.

22. Handen BL, Johnson CR, Lubetsky M. Efficacy of methylphenidate among children with autism and symptoms of attention-deficit hyperactivity disorder. *J Autism Dev Disord.* 2000;30:245–255.

23. Research Units on Pediatric Psychopharmacology Autism Network. Randomized, controlled, crossover trial of methylphenidate in pervasive developmental disorders with hyperactivity. *Arch Gen Psychiatry.* 2005;62:1266–1274.

24. Aman MG. Management of hyperactivity and other acting-out problems in autism spectrum disorder. *Semin Pediatr Neurol.* 2004;11:225–228.

25. Fankhauser MP, Karumanchi VC, German ML, Yates A, Karumanchi SD. A double-blind, placebo-controlled study of the efficacy of transdermal clonidine in autism. *J Clin Psychiatry.* 1992;53:77–82.

26. Jaselskis CA, Cook EH, Fletcher E, Leventhal BL. Clonidine treatment of hyperactive and impulsive children with autistic disorder. *J Clin Psychopharmacol.* 1992;12:322–327.

27. Scahill L, Aman MG, McDougle CJ, et al. A prospective open trial of guanfacine in children with pervasive developmental disorders. Research Units on Pediatric Psychopharmacology (RUPP) Autism Network. *J Child Adolesc Psychopharmacol.* 2006;16:589–598.

28. Posey DJ, Puntney JI, Sasher TM, Kem DL, McDougle CJ. Guanfacine treatment of hyperactivity and inattention in pervasive developmental disorders: a retrospective analysis of 80 cases. *J Child Adolesc Psychopharmacol.* 2004;14:233–241.

29. Reed MD, Findling RL. Overview of current management of sleep disturbances in children: I—pharmacotherapy. *Curr Ther Res.* 2002;63(Suppl. B):B18–B37.

30. Mehta UC, Patel I, Castello FV. EEG sedation for children with autism. *J Dev Behav Pediatr.* 2004;25:102–104.

31. Ingrassia A, Turk J. The use of clonidine for severe and intractable sleep problems in children with neurodevelopmental disorders: a case series. *Eur Child Adolesc Psychiatry.* 2005;14:34–40.

32. Posey DJ, Guenin KD, Kohn AE, Swiezy NB, McDougle CJ. A naturalistic open-label study of mirtazapine in autistic and other pervasive developmental disorders. *J Child Adolesc Psychopharmacol.* 2001;11:267–277.

33. Jou RJ, Handen BL, Hardan AY. Retrospective assessment of atomoxetine in children and adolescents with pervasive developmental disorders. *J Child Adolesc Psychopharmacol.* 2005;15:325–330.

34. Posey DJ, Wiegand RE, Wilkerson J, Maynard M, Stigler KA, McDougle CJ. Open-label atomoxetine for attention-deficit/hyperactivity disorder symptoms associated with high-functioning pervasive developmental disorders. *J Child Adolesc Psychopharmacol.* 2006;16:599–610.

35. Arnold LE, Aman MG, Cook AM, et al. Atomoxetine for hyperactivity in autism spectrum disorders: placebo-controlled crossover pilot trial. *J Am Acad Child Adolesc Psychiatry.* 2006;45:1196–1205.

36. Rugino TA, Samsock TC. Levetiracetam in autistic children: an open-label study. *J Dev Behav Pediatr.* 2002;23:225–230.

37. Hardan AY, Jou RJ, Handen BL. A retrospective assessment of topiramate in children and adolescents with pervasive developmental disorders. *J Child Adolesc Psychopharmacol.* 2004;14:426–432.

38. Connor DF, Ozbayrak KR, Benjamin S, Ma Y, Fletcher KE. A pilot study of nadolol for overt aggression in developmentally delayed individuals. *J Am Acad Child Adolesc Psychiatry.* 1997;36:826–834.

39. Ratey JJ, Mikkelsen E, Sorgi P, et al. Autism: the treatment of aggressive behaviors. *J Clin Psychopharmacol.* 1987;7:35–41.

40. Bostic JQ, Rho Y. Target-symptom psychopharmacology: between the forest and the trees. *Child Adolesc Psychiatr Clin N Am.* 2006;15:289–302.

41. Stigler KA, Posey DJ, McDougle CJ. Ramelteon for insomnia in two youths with autistic disorder. *J Child Adolesc Psychopharmacol.* 2006;16:631–636.

42. Owens JA, Babcock D, Blumer J, et al. The use of pharmacotherapy in the treatment of pediatric insomnia in primary care: rational approaches—a consensus meeting summary. *J Clin Sleep Med.* 2005;1:49–59.

43. Buitelaar JK, van der Gaag RJ, van der Hoeven J. Buspirone in the management of anxiety and irritability in children with pervasive developmental disorders: results of an open-label study. *J Clin Psychiatry.* 1998;59:56–59.

44. Myers SM, Challman TD. Psychopharmacology: an approach to management in autism and intellectual disabilities. In: Accardo PJ, ed. *Capute & Accardo's Neurodevelopmental Disabilities in Infancy and Childhood: Vol I. Neurodevelopmental Diagnosis and Treatment.* 3rd ed. Baltimore, MD: Paul H Brookes; 2008:577–614.

45. Kowatch RA, DelBello MD. Pediatric bipolar disorder: emerging diagnostic and treatment approaches. *Child Adolesc Psychiatr Clin N Am.* 2006;15:73–108.

46. Vitiello B. An update on publicly funded multisite trials in pediatric psychopharmacology. *Child Adolesc Psychiatr Clin N Am.* 2006;15:1–12.

47. Owley T, Walton L, Salt J, et al. An open-label trial of escitalopram in pervasive developmental disorders. *J Am Acad Child Adolesc Psychiatry.* 2005;44:343–348.

48. Kerbeshian J, Burd L, Fisher W. Lithium carbonate in the treatment of two patients with infantile autism and atypical bipolar symptomatology. *J Clin Psychopharmacol.* 1987;7:401–405.

49. Steingard R, Biederman J. Lithium responsive manic-like symptoms in two individuals with autism and mental retardation. *J Am Acad Child Adolesc Psychiatry.* 1987;26:932–935.

19 Complementary and Alternative Medicine

Complementary and alternative medicine (CAM) is a group of diverse medical and health care systems, practices, and products that are not generally considered part of conventional medicine. According to a nationwide government survey released in December 2008, approximately 38% of U.S. adults aged 18 years and older and approximately 12% of children use some form of CAM. Such CAM treatments are becoming widely used as an adjunct to conventional medical treatment for many conditions, including autism spectrum disorders (ASD).

Brumback, in his review of the excellent text, Ernst's *Trick or Treatment: The Undeniable Facts about Alternative Medicine* (1), states that "on January 1, 2010, a Google search of the Internet using the term 'alternative medicine' revealed 16 million Web sites: the first site listed is by the National Center for Complementary and Alternative Medicine of the National Institutes of Health demonstrating the United States government approval of this movement, which is the 21st Century version of the medical quackery and charlatanism that pervaded the Middle Ages through the early 20th Century" (1–10).

A recent study was conducted in 14 major metropolitan areas in the United States and Canada to determine the frequency of CAM treatments in a large ASD registry and identify factors associated with the use of CAM treatments (11). Researchers found that among 1,200 children and teenagers with a diagnosis along the autism spectrum, fully 21% reported CAM use. Of these, by far and away the most common CAM use was dietary modification. Of the modified diets, gluten-free and casein-free were the most common. "Other" diets included soy-free; milk-, lactose-, or dairy-free; dye-free; and specific allergen-free. The most common "treatment" was the use of a wide variety of vitamins and probiotics, and used by 12% across the autism spectrum of diagnoses. Among other observations, it was noted that children with gastrointestinal problems were more likely to be on any CAM treatment and were specifically more likely to have been treated with special diets, digestive enzymes, other vitamins, or probiotics.

One of the most important findings in a large multisite study was that CAM treatments for children and teenagers with an ASD are almost double that in children in the United States generally (12), revealing the exceptional vulnerability of individuals with an ASD diagnosis. It is obvious from all these data that much more vigorous and robust, peer-reviewed, and double-blinded studies before practitioners recommend CAM therapies, which are often expensive, useless, and at times, dangerous. As Ernst (13) concisely states in a recent editorial, there are several fallacies in either whole-heartedly embracing or rejecting CAM:

1. *If it's natural, it's safe:* There is nothing natural about high doses of vitamins or about acupuncture needles in children's tongues. To state that a product or procedure is natural and therefore safe is intrinsically dangerous.
2. *CAM defies science:* To the contrary, such statements clearly indicate how poorly understood is the scientific method and what it can achieve.
3. *There is no evidence:* To the contrary, there is typically *some* evidence, but the evidence often negates the claim of the practitioners. Additionally, to state that a particular therapy is not harmful does not make it necessarily helpful.
4. *CAM saves money:* Indeed, if this were the case, most insurance companies would be insisting on CAM prior to conventional and evidence-based medical practices. However, evidence consistently shows that CAM is typically more expensive than evidence-based approaches.
5. *Anecdotes top evidence:* It is important not to dismiss reports of improvement in the context of any therapy; however, it is exceptionally misleading to associate causal improvement when

only a temporal relationship exists. A host of factors may contribute to improvement; in the absence of blinded and peer-reviewed data, anecdotal evidence is among the most dangerous upon which to rely.

6. *The "establishment" wants to suppress CAM:* Despite the popularity of this argument, there is no evidence that it is true. On the contrary, there is plenty of evidence to show that doctors are more than willing to adopt any treatment that helps their patients and that "big pharma" takes little—if any—notice of CAM (14).

ABOVE ALL, DO NO HARM

Those therapies which to date have either inadequate or no basis in scientific or peer-reviewed research specific to ASD should be avoided. In the opinion of many respected researchers in the field, that list to date would include, but not necessarily be limited to, the following:

1. Acupuncture
2. Cranial sacral therapy
3. Chiropractics
4. Chelation therapy
5. Dietary changes, specifically soy-free; milk-, lactose-, or dairy-free; dye-free; and specific allergen-free, in the absence of formal assessment by well-trained pediatric allergy-immunologists
6. Megavitamin supplementation
7. Hyperbaric chamber use
8. Oxygen supplementation
9. Chronic use of antiviral agents, such as acyclovir, or other antimicrobials in the absence of documented active infection in an otherwise immune-competent individual

In summary, pediatricians continue to represent an important protective barrier against the use of desperate unfounded therapies. Even in the absence of physical harm, many of these "therapies" are exorbitantly expensive, and not only provide no benefit, but also permanently financially damage a young family's ability to provide for the child's long-term educational and therapeutic needs. As parents bring in material for the pediatrician's input, careful listening to the family's concern and review of the materials with further research as necessary are important. However, in the absence of any robust data to recommend a specific CAM, it is in the child's best interest to avoid what are often unsubstantiated, expensive, and potentially dangerous therapies.

REFERENCES

1. Brumback RA. Book review: Simon Singh and Edzard Ernst trick or treatment: the undeniable facts about alternative medicine. *J Child Neurol.* 2010;25:651.
2. Singh S, Ernst E. *Trick or Treatment: The Undeniable Facts about Alternative Medicine.* New York: WW Norton & Company; 2008.
3. Brock P. *Charlatan: America's Most Dangerous Huckster, the Man Who Pursued Him, and the Age of Flimflam.* New York: Crown Publishers; 2008.
4. Brumback RA. Charlatan: America's most dangerous huckster, the man who pursued him, and the age of flimflam [book review]. *J Child Neurol.* 2009;24:1574–1577.
5. Offit PA. *Autism's False Prophets: Bad Science, Risky Medicine, and the Search for a Cure.* New York: Columbia University Press; 2008.
6. Brumback RA. Autism's false prophets: bad science, risky medicine, and the search for a cure [book review]. *J Child Neurol.* 2009;24:251–252.
7. Goldacre B. *Bad Science.* London: Fourth Estate; 2009.
8. Smith RL. *At Your Own Risk: The Case against Chiropractic.* New York: Trident Press; 1969.
9. Huber PW. *Galileo's Revenge: Junk Science in the Courtroom.* New York: Basic Books; 1993.
10. Wootton D. *Bad Medicine: Doctors Doing Harm Since Hippocrates.* New York: Oxford University Press; 2007.

11. Coury D, Jones, Klatka K, Winklosky B, Perrin JM. (2009). Healthcare for children with autism: the Autism Treatment Network. *Curr Opin Pediatr.* 2009;21(6), 828–32.

12. Christon, LM, Mackintosh VH, Myers BJ. Use of complementary and alternative medicine (CAM) treatments by parents of children with autism spectrum disorders. *Res Autism Spectr Disord.* 2010;4(2): 249–259.

13. Ernst E. How the public is being misled about complementary and alternative medicine. *J R Soc Med.* 2008;101:528–530.

14. Thompson Coon J, Pittler M, Ernst E. Herb-drug interactions: survey of leading pharmaceutical/herbal companies. *Arch Intern Med.* 2003;163:1371.

For more in-depth reading about CAM, the reader is urged to review the following excellent texts:

1. Ernst E, Pittler MH, Wider B, Boddy K. *The Desktop Guide to Complementary and Alternative Medicine.* 2nd ed. Edinburgh, UK: Elsevier Mosby; 2006.

Section Four:

Autism Spectrum Disorders and the Public School

SAMPLE CASE

Tommy is a 7-year-old handsome, very verbal, but socially very odd, child. His family brought him to their primary care provider (PCP) for evaluation. The history revealed that the child made straight As in his math and language classes. However, he struggled to get through any of the noncore subjects, such as music or art. He would spin, run, talk incessantly, make strange repetitive noises, and be generally disruptive. Further, the other children tended to avoid him, although this did not seem to be a concern to him. During Tommy examination, his spoken language was notably sophisticated and closer to a much older child's use of vocabulary. However, he had no control over his voice modulation, tending to shout and get directly into the faces of the family and the examiner. Further, he was exceptionally well versed on all the movies of Robin Williams, being able to recite the entire dialogues at a time. The remainder of his examination was largely normal. A referral to speech therapy was made in order to enhance his pragmatic speech skills, as well as a referral to a child psychologist to start social skills coaching. Because it was going to take literally half a year to obtain psychometric testing, the family was provided a prescription with the diagnosis of "Asperger's Syndrome; please evaluate," written on it.

Tommy's parents presented a diagnosis along with the services requested by his physician. With the script in hand, they believed that the school would finally provide him with the services he needed to be successful. They were dismayed when they were told that because of his excellent grades, he did not qualify for either services or even psychometric testing. Indeed, the school refused to recognize the physician-generated diagnosis of an autistic spectrum disorder (ASD), specifically Asperger's syndrome, because Tommy did not demonstrate academic need (i.e., failing or near-failing). The family was informed that a medical diagnosis does not automatically entitle a student to special education services; rather, eligibility is based on an educational determination of a disability. Frustrated, the family returned to the physician's office for further assistance. The family was put in touch with a local school advocate to see if additional services could be obtained because of his Asperger's syndrome diagnosis.

ALL ON ONE TEAM

The nature of the complexity of autistic diagnoses makes finding solutions for classroom services particularly challenging. The PCP has not only the opportunity but oftentimes the ethical duty to facilitate such services if at all possible. However, sometimes navigating the public school requirements can feel intimidating and confusing to families as well as health professionals who are seeking to streamline the process on their behalf. However, there are ways in which obtaining the needed assessment and services from the public schools can be done, and in a way that maximizes a sense of team spirit among educators, clinicians, and families.

SCREENING GUIDELINES FOR THE PCP

Accurate diagnosis of an ASD requires multidisciplinary involvement among professionals, families, schools, and service agencies. An ASD affects numerous developmental domains; therefore, it requires numerous areas of specialties (e.g., health care, speech, occupational/physical therapy, behavior, education, and psychology). An advantage of collaborative involvement is the reduction and avoidance of a duplication of services.

The PCP is often the initial point of contact for a family that has concerns for their child. Many parents with children with autistic symptoms suspect that something is wrong by the time their child is 18 months old and often seek help by the time they are 2. The PCP is essential to the diagnostic process with regard to appropriate referral through medical, school, or community settings, as well as being a liaison and advocate for the child and family.

The American Academy of Pediatrics (1–3) recommends that all children should be screened for ASD at 18 months and 24 months, regardless of whether there are any signs or concerns about a child's developmental process. The standardized guidelines developed for the diagnosis of autism involve two levels of screening for autism. Level 1 screening, which should be performed for all children coming to a physician for well-child checkups during their first 2 years of life, should check the following developmental deficits:

- No babbling, pointing, or gesturing by age 12 months
- No single words spoken by age 16 months
- No two-word spontaneous (nonecholalic, or not merely repeating the sounds of others) expressions by age 24 months
- Loss of any language or social skills at any age
- No eye contact at 3 to 4 months

Level 2 screening should be performed if a child is identified in the first level of screening as developmentally delayed and is a more in-depth diagnosis and evaluation that can differentiate autism from other developmental disorders. The second level of screening may include more formal diagnostic procedures by clinicians skilled in diagnosing autism, including medical history, neurologic evaluation, genetic testing, metabolic testing, electrophysiologic testing (i.e., computerized tomography scan, magnetic resonance imaging, positron emission tomography scan), psychometric and/or psychological testing, among others (1,2).

BENEFIT OF EARLY DIAGNOSIS

Timely referral, coordination of evaluation, and early diagnosis enhance long-term outcomes for individuals with autism and lead to more efficient service delivery through locally-, state-, and federally funded programs. Diagnoses provide a common language and framework among specialists, providers, and families (4).

AUTISM DIAGNOSIS IN THE PRIMARY CARE SETTING

Health care providers will often use a questionnaire or other screening instrument to gather information about a child's development and behavior. Some screening instruments rely solely on parent observations, whereas others rely on a combination of parent, teacher, and/or doctor observations. If screening instruments indicate the possibility of ASD, a more comprehensive evaluation is strongly recommended. As noted previously, a comprehensive evaluation requires a multidisciplinary team, such as a psychologist, neurologist, psychiatrist, diagnostician, and speech therapist.

There is no single test that provides enough information to be used as the sole basis for the diagnosis of autism. A diagnosis of autism should be based on the criteria in the American Psychiatric Association's *Diagnostic and Statistical Manual of Mental Disorders, 4th Edition-Text Revision* (DSM-IV-TR; 5) or the most current edition of this manual. Although there are alternative diagnostic models, to date they lack a formal research base and have not gained acceptance among developmental specialists.

COMPONENTS OF A DIAGNOSTIC EVALUATION

- Background information
  - Parent/caregiver interview
    - Health history: prenatal and perinatal histories; medical history; review of systems (e.g., hearing, vision, and gastrointestinal)
  - Developmental and behavioral history
    - Aggression, fears, separation anxiety, and fearless behavior
  - Family medical and mental health history
  - Assessment of family resources and needs
- Medical evaluation
  - General physical and neurodevelopmental examination
  - Laboratory tests
  - Genetic testing
  - Sensory evaluation (vision and hearing)
- Direct behavior observation
  - Observe interaction with the family and other familiar/unfamiliar adults
  - Speech, movement, eye contact, etc.
  - Stereotypic behaviors (e.g., hand flapping, flicking, body rocking, and head banging)
    - [*Note:* Excessive motor stereotypic behavior is associated with greater degrees of cognitive impairment (e.g., mental retardation) and not just in the ASD population.]
- Cognitive assessment (for differential diagnosis determination and intervention planning)
- Adaptive functioning
  - Communication
    - Receptive and expressive language
    - Pragmatic language/social communication/reciprocal communication
    - Nonverbal communication (eye contact, use of gaze, and gestures)
    - Echolalia
  - Socialization/social–emotional functioning
  - Fine and gross motor development, coordination, gait, and motor planning
  - Daily living/self-help skills—hygiene, toileting, eating, and dressing
    - [*Note:* Uneven skill profiles of children with ASD are common; motor and daily living/self-help skills are often relatively better than socialization and communication.]
- Sensory processing: hyper- or hyposensitivities to foods, smells, textures, sounds, etc.
- Behavioral functioning
  - Serious behavioral difficulties can affect the child's safety, interfere with family functioning, and limit the child's and family's participation with extended family and the community (e.g., church and dining at restaurants)

The previous items are for children from birth to 5 years. Children older than 6 years also need these components of an evaluation, as well as the following additional measures:

- Record review
- Direct child evaluation: interview and observation in different environments
- Mental health assessment/psychiatric functioning
- Achievement testing, if academic concerns exist
- Behavior
  - Mood, aggression, and withdrawal
  - Interests and activities
    - Restricted/narrowly defined interests
    - Ritualistic or compulsive behaviors
- Social competence and functioning
- Attention and concentration, impulsivity, and regulation of activity level

WHEN TO REFER TO AUTISM SPECIALTY CLINICS

As noted previously in this chapter, the second level of screening for autism involves formal diagnostic procedures, including neurologic, psychological, and psychometric testing, as well as genetic, metabolic, and electrophysiologic testing (1,2).

You can find these multidisciplinary services for your patients in an autism specialty clinic. Finding a specialty clinic for your patients can be a daunting task in many parts of the country; however, the benefits outweigh the initial time spent locating and developing a collaborative relationship. This involves determining the required referral method and creating a collaborative effort that can reduce your patient's referral waiting time.

SPECIALISTS IN ASD

Individuals qualified for diagnosing ASD should have completed graduate and/or postgraduate studies in psychology, education, and/or child development, with emphasis on developmental disabilities (e.g., autism and neurodevelopmental disorders). Experience in clinical, educational, and/or treatment settings that include children with ASD is critical. A skilled diagnostician integrates findings from previous evaluations and observations from parents and others familiar with the child (e.g., speech/language pathologists and teachers), along with determining appropriate evaluative measures.

Training and clinical experience in the diagnosis and treatment of ASD or fellowship in a credentialed medical training program in pediatrics, child neurology, or child psychiatry is critical for residents and fellows. Clinical experience with the variability within the population with ASD is paramount for PCPs.

STABILITY OF DIAGNOSIS AND THE NEED FOR REEVALUATION

Children are being referred and diagnosed with ASD at earlier ages. Annual follow-up evaluations are recommended for children younger than 5 years because of the instability of diagnosis at very young ages (e.g., 2 years and younger). It is possible for a child to be diagnosed with ASD at age 2; however, the diagnosis may change at age 4 or 5 years because of intervention and developmental growth.

AUTISM DIAGNOSIS IN AN EDUCATIONAL MODEL

A medical diagnosis of autism is determined by the physician on the basis of the assessment of symptoms and diagnostic tests. It is often made in accordance to the *Diagnostic and Statistical Manual of Mental Disorders* (DSM-IV-TR) of the American Psychological Association (APA, 2000; 5). An educational diagnosis, referred to as a determination, is made by a multidisciplinary team and typically includes a diagnostician, speech and language pathologist, school psychologist, special education teacher, and the parents/guardians.

The results of the evaluation determine if a student is eligible for special education and related services under Individuals with Disabilities Education Act (IDEA; 6). In contrast to the variety of medical disorders a patient may be diagnosed with by a physician, the education system is limited to the following disability categories:

- Mental retardation (aka cognitive impairment or disability)
- Hearing impairment (including deafness)
- Visual impairment (including blindness)
- Deaf-blindness
- Speech or language impairment
- Emotional disturbance

- Orthopedic impairment
- Autism
- Traumatic brain injury
- Other health impaired
- Specific learning disability
- Multiple disabilities

An educational determination for services is based on the impact of the condition on the student's learning. Unlike a diagnosis for disorders such as diabetes and epilepsy, a diagnosis of autism can be made through the school without the need for a medical diagnosis. Therefore, a student may have a diagnosis by a physician, but the multidisciplinary team may determine that the condition does not affect the child's ability to be involved in and progress in the general education curriculum. If this is the case, the student will not be provided special services under IDEA (6,7).

Multidisciplinary evaluations within a public school setting may be administered before age 3 for early childhood programs and/or for children who are 3 years old or older for special education services for programs such as preschool program for children with disabilities (PPCD), prekindergarten, and head start.

Assessments will differ because of the age, ability level, and needs of the child, and will include the assessment of preacademic and academic skills, self-help and adaptive skills, communication, socialization, sensory regulation, motivation and reinforcement, behavior, fine and gross motor, play and leisure, as well as cognition. For older students, prevocational and vocational skills are also assessed (8). Reevaluations are required to be conducted every 3 years (triennial) or more frequently if needed (9).

INDIVIDUALIZED FAMILY SERVICE PLAN AND INDIVIDUALIZED EDUCATION PROGRAM

The multidisciplinary and comprehensive assessment determines if a child meets eligibility for special education services and provides guidance in the development of an individualized family service plan (IFSP) for children younger than 3 years and individualized education program (IEP) for children/students ages 3 to 21. IEPs for students with ASD should have goals and objectives designed to promote the development of independent living, academic skills, and appropriate social behaviors and skills (10).

The IEP team can include individuals outside of school personnel who have knowledge or special expertise regarding the child and/or the disorder. This is at the discretion of the parent/guardian or the agency (11).

COGNITIVE ASSESSMENT

Accurate assessment of skills is often difficult to determine in children with autism because of variable skills, such as language and level of participation during the assessments. It is important to note that although mental retardation is a common comorbid disorder, not all children with ASD (e.g., PDD-NOS and Asperger's syndrome) have low cognitive functioning.

COMMUNICATION

Verbal and nonverbal communicative skills need to be assessed. How a child expresses him-/herself nonverbally (e.g., gestures such as pointing to show or request and item, eye gaze, and expressions) is just as important as how he/she communicates through sounds and words. Hearing acuity should also be assessed. Children with autism often display language that is rote, repetitive (i.e., echolalic), or lack contextual meaning.

SOCIAL INTERACTION

One of the primary components of a diagnosis of autism includes an individual's restricted ability in forming relationships; therefore, assessment of the child's ability of social initiation (e.g., eye contact, playing with other children, lack of interest in being held, and invading other's personal space), imitation (e.g., imitating other's actions, such as parent cleaning or shaving), and isolation, as well as reciprocity in games and communication (verbal and nonverbal), and attachment to the parent/caregiver.

BEHAVIOR PATTERNS AND RESPONSES TO THE ENVIRONMENT

Determination of restricted, repetitive, and stereotyped patterns of behavior, interest, and activities is paramount in the assessment and intervention of a child exhibiting characteristics of autism. Problematic behavior and patterns (e.g., aggressive, disruptive, and frustration tolerance), along with sensory issues (e.g., clothing, food textures, temperature, and noise), are common problems in children with ASD. Determining patterns and triggers can assist families and schools, and help with implementation of successful intervention plans.

Repetitive motor and verbal behaviors can include movements such as flapping hands, jumping up and down, rocking, spinning, banging heads, and repetitive finger movements. These behaviors are often most evident when the child is anxious, excited, or upset.

FUNCTIONAL BEHAVIORAL ASSESSMENTS

Another type of assessment within a school setting is the functional behavioral assessment (FBA). Students with autism may experience significant behavioral problems, often due to frustration and anxiety, which are related to their difficulties with communication, sensory regulation, and/or social interactions. Functional assessments use a variety of ways to gather information (e.g., observations, school faculty/staff and parent input, checklists/ratings, psychological assessment, and functional analysis).

An FBA analyzes an individual student's disruptive behaviors in order to identify appropriate interventions. The "ABC" analysis of the FBA includes the identification of the *a*ntecedent conditions that precede the undesirable *b*ehavior (e.g., transitions and changes in routine), and the determined *c*onsequences to reduce/eliminate the behavior. Using the results of the FBA, a behavior intervention plan (BIP) is developed that includes positive behavioral supports or strategies (e.g., rewarding, ignoring, and redirecting) intended to change the student's behavior.

REFERENCES

1. American Academy of Pediatrics, Committee on Children with Disabilities. Developmental surveillance and screening in young children. *Pediatrics.* 2001;108:192–195.
2. Johnson CP, Myers SM; Council on Children with Disabilities, American Academy of Pediatrics. Identification and evaluation of children with autism spectrum disorders. *Pediatrics.* 2007;120:1183–1215.
3. American Academy of Pediatrics; Council on Children with Disabilities, Section on Developmental Behavioral Pediatrics, Bright Futures Steering Committee, Medical Home Initiatives for Children with Special Needs Project Advisory Committee. Identifying infants and young children with developmental disorders: an algorithm for developmental surveillance and screening. *Pediatrics.* 2006;118: 405–420. [Published correction appears in *Pediatrics.* 2006;118:1808–1809.]
4. Committee on Children with Disabilities. The pediatrician's role in the diagnosis and management of autistic spectrum disorder in children. *Pediatrics.* 2001;107:1221–1226.
5. American Psychiatric Association. *Diagnostic and Statistical Manual of Mental Disorders.* 4th ed. *Text Revision (DSM-IV-TR).* Washington, DC: American Psychiatric Publishing; 2000.
6. Individuals with Disabilities Education Act of 2004, P.L. 108-446, 20 U.S.C. §1400 et seq.

7. Hawkins SC. (2009). Medical diagnosis vs. educational determination: a distinction that makes a difference. http://www.ttac.vt.edu/autism/documents/E-News_January_09.pdf. Retrieved June 15, 2010.

8. Office of Superintendent of Public Instruction (OSPI) (2008). *The Educational Aspects of Autism Spectrum Disorders.* Olympia, WA. http://www.k12.wa.us. Retrieved March 1, 2009.

9. Sattler JM. *Assessment of Children.* Revised and updated 3rd ed. San Diego, CA: Jerome M. Sattler, Publisher, Inc; 1992.

10. National Education Association (NEA) (2006). *The puzzle of autism.* http://www.nea.org/assets/docs/autismpuzzle.pdf. Retrieved May 10, 2010.

11. Turnbull HR, Wilcox BL, Stowe MJ. Brief overview of special education law with focus on autism. *J Autism Dev Disord.* 2002;32(5):479–493.

21

Medical Statements That May Help Children with Autistic Spectrum Disorders in the Classroom

SAMPLE CASE

Cathy's mother requested and received a letter of diagnosis from her child's physician that noted the child's current diagnosis, date of diagnosis, and prescribed medications, as well as a request to the school to complete a comprehensive evaluation and provide Cathy with the support services that would appropriately address her needs as a child with autism. Cathy's mother also provided the school with a well-organized and comprehensive compilation of chronological data (medical history, interventions/therapies, evaluations, and behaviors). She braced herself for a struggle with the school, but was very pleased that the school completed the evaluation and determined Cathy to be eligible for special education services.

HOW MEDICAL LETTERS FROM TREATING PRIMARY CARE PROVIDERS HELP

Referral to early intervention, school, and/or other services can often be facilitated by a letter from the child's physician or specialist. This can be incredibly helpful for families as well as schools to clearly understand how potentially serious a child's or teenager's situation may be. As noted in the Chapter 20, a medical diagnosis differs from an educational determination; however, schools are required by law to consider the professional recommendations of doctors. When a doctor sends a letter of recommendation requesting educational interventions, behavioral, therapeutic, or medical interventions to be done at school, their expertise should be considered and implemented to the degree that the child can derive the greatest benefit from the educational system.

This chapter includes examples of letters that parents should provide to their child's school requesting an evaluation (e.g., psychological and educational testing, a speech and language evaluation, occupational therapy assessment, and behavioral analysis; see Appendix E).

Parents/guardians should be strongly encouraged to keep records about their child, including the following:

- Professionals seen (date, time, reason for contact, result, and contact information)
- Letters, e-mails, and faxes from the school and other professionals/service providers
- Evaluations and progress notes from the school and outside professionals (e.g., therapists)
- School documents (e.g., individual education plans, samples of school work, report cards, school conferences, and disciplinary notices)
- Additionally, parents should be encouraged to create a document that includes developmental history, personal observations about difficulties and strengths, illnesses, behaviors, family medical histories, and so on

Letters from you and the parents should be submitted to a school administrator, such as the principal or the special education administrator. The letters should be succinct, typically one page. Counsel the patient's parents to use neutral language and not angry or accusatory statements in their letter. The letters can be hand-delivered, but a copy of the letters should be stamped with the date and signed by the school personnel that received the letters (e.g., secretary).

It is preferable to send the letters by certified mail with a return confirmation receipt. If the letters have been mailed and no response has been received in 10 days, the parents should contact the administrator to determine the delay in a response (4).

The family should receive a written response that includes a consent or denial of an evaluation plan. If it is denied, then a rationale must be provided. Once the consent form for assessment is signed by the parents/guardians and returned to the school, the school has 60 days to evaluate the child unless the state has set its own time frame (4). If a school does not respond to parents' request for an evaluation, they should contact their state education agency (5,6).

SUMMARY

In our experience, public schools are typically eager for communication from both parents and primary care providers (PCPs). Having a standardized approach to providing needed medical diagnoses proactively to the school can be exceptionally helpful in facilitating services specific to the needs of the student, as well as setting an excellent precedent for good communication between all parties as long as the child is enrolled in the public school system. Because many children with severe disabilities are often served until age 21, having good documentation from both the parents and the PCP helps pave the way for adult services at the end of a child's public school training.

REFERENCES

1. Learning Disabilities about.com. *Referral letter.* http://www.learningdisabilities.about.com/library/ regulations/referralletter.doc. Retrieved July 11, 2010.
2. Ferguson S, Ripley S. (2000). *Special Education and Related Services: Communicating Through Letter Writing.* http://kidsource.com/NICHCY/letter.dis.k12.4.1.html
3. Los Angeles Unified School District. *The special education process.* http://sped.lausd.net/sepg2s/ pg2_gettingstarted.htm. May 2010 was the last update. Original publication date is not listed
4. National Dissemination Center for Children with Disabilities (NICHCY). (2009). *Your Child's Evaluation.* http://www.nichcy.org/InformationResources/Documents/ NICHCY%20PUBS/ bp1.pdf. Retrieved June 23, 2010.
5. American Academy of Child & Adolescent Psychiatry. (2008). *Services in School for Children with Special Needs: What Parents Need to Know.* http://www.aacap.org/cs/root/facts_for_families/services_in_ school_for_children_with_ special_needs_what_parents_need_to_know. Retrieved June 23, 2010.
6. Great Schools. *Special Education: An Overview.* http://www.greatschools.org/special-education/ legal-rights/special-education-evaluation-an-overview.gs?content=666. Retrieved July 28, 2010.

22

Finding Ways to Help Families Navigate the Public School System

SAMPLE CASE

Cindy was diagnosed with autism at age 3. Her school district provided placement in their half-day preschool special education program with integrated (in class) speech service provision. After 4 months, Cindy's parents believed that her behavior had regressed and her stereotypical mannerisms had increased in intensity. The parents believed that the regressions were due to the school's program not being designed to meet Cindy's unique needs. After presenting a letter to the school principal requesting additional services and a move to another school, the school district responded that she was receiving appropriate services and a placement change was unnecessary. The parents subsequently retained the services of an advocate to assist them in navigating the special education system to get the services Cindy needed.

NAVIGATING THE PUBLIC SCHOOLS: HOW PRIMARY CARE PHYSICIANS HELP

Parents and schools often conflict on services for students. Parents naturally seek services that they believe are *best* for their children, whereas schools are obligated to only provide services that are deemed *appropriate* for children with special needs (1). Complaints against school districts predominantly result over issues concerning referrals for assessments, evaluations, individual education plan (IEP) development and implementation, lack of educational progress, and the provision of related services such as speech, occupation, and/or physical therapy.

Under the *Individuals with Disabilities Education Act* (IDEA; 2), resolutions over special education disagreements between parents and school districts include mediation, formal complaints, and due process hearings. IDEA requires that special education disputes must proceed through these levels, including appeals, before either party files a lawsuit in civil court. Parents should be encouraged to initially seek informal resolution by meeting with the principal and/or special education administrator of their child's school or filing a complaint with the local school board through the district superintendent.

When conflicts cannot be resolved through the IEP process or through school or district administrators, the state government's special education department can assist through consultation or mediation services. If this is not successful, then filing a formal special education complaint is the next step. The state education agency (SEA) will provide information about the process, the parents' rights, resources, and the information to assist in resolving the conflict through alternative means (e.g., mediation, due process hearing; 3).

A typical process for the SEA is to have an investigator review the complaint and may contact the parents to discuss the issue(s). A letter will then be sent to the parents and the school district, stating the IDEA issues related to the allegations, the procedures to be followed, and options to resolve the issue(s). Self-investigations and/or resolutions by the school district may be the next step or a comprehensive investigation will be completed with a formal report by the SEA being provided to the parents/guardians and the school district. The formal report will explain the process, the facts uncovered during the investigation, a listing of any violations found, and corrective actions to be taken by the school district. The parents/guardians and also the school district can appeal decisions made in the investigation.

MEDIATION

In *mediation*, the parties gather to discuss the presenting problems and attempt to arrive at a resolution. The no-cost, voluntary mediation process is managed by a qualified and impartial mediator between the parents and the school district administrators (2–5). The SEA maintains a list of qualified mediators who are knowledgeable in special education laws and regulations and related services. These mediators are selected on a random, rotational, or other impartial basis. Unlike situations with a judge or an arbitrator, the decision-making authority rests with the parties. If the matter is successfully resolved, the parties create a written mediation agreement, including the settlement terms and conditions, which is enforceable in court (1,3,4).

Following IDEA (2) rules and regulations, the mediation process must be voluntary on the part of the parties and is not used to deny or delay a parent's right to a due process hearing. The state bears the cost of the mediation process. The mediation process is confidential and discussions that occur during the mediation process cannot be used as evidence in any subsequent due process hearings or civil proceedings. It is not required that the parents enlist the services of a special education attorney for a mediation hearing, although consulting with an attorney beforehand would be strongly recommended (6).

DUE PROCESS HEARINGS

A *due process hearing* is similar to a hearing in civil court. Presumably, a school district will send its attorney to the hearing; therefore, parents should also be represented by an attorney that specializes in special education law. The plaintiff (e.g., parents) provides an opening statement with details of the allegations against the defendant (e.g., school district). Both the parties are provided an opportunity to cross-examine any witnesses that testify during the hearing. The plaintiff has the burden of proof in a due process hearing, and both the parties must prove that any allegations presented are factual. Documentation must support the allegations, and often it includes the child's cumulative records, including the special education files (e.g., referrals for assessment, evaluation results from school/private evaluators and state assessments, IEPs, progress reports, discipline reports, and attendance records) (1).

An *impartial hearing officer* (IHO), also known as an administrative law judge, is an expert in administrative law who presides over *special education due process hearings*. They can be attorneys or educators with advanced legal training. Decisions rendered by IHOs are legally binding on *parties in the dispute*. Both the parties may *appeal the ruling* if reasonable evidence is presented that the IHO made an error or that additional evidence has surfaced that may affect the outcome of the case (1).

A parent or agency must request a due process hearing within 2 years of the date the parent or agency knew or should have known about the alleged action that forms the basis of the due process complaint. This timeline does not apply if specific misrepresentations by the local educational agency (LEA) indicated that it had resolved the problem forming the basis of the due process complaint or if the LEA withheld information from the parent (2,4).

The LEA must convene a meeting with the parent and the member(s) of the IEP team within 15 days of receiving notice of the parent's due process complaint and prior to the initiation of a due processing hearing. The meeting must not include an attorney of the LEA unless the parent is accompanied by an attorney. This meeting allows the LEA to have the opportunity to resolve the dispute that is the basis for the due process complaint. If the LEA has not resolved the due process complaint to the satisfaction of the parent within 30 days of the receipt of the due process complaint, the due process hearing may occur (4). If there are unsatisfactory results of the due process hearing, then a lawsuit in civil court is the next step.

PROFESSIONAL DISABILITY ADVOCATES

Disability advocates can assist parents in working more effectively with school personnel in the planning and implementation of effective educational programs for their child. They can assist the parents through the IEP process by reviewing the child's school records and can attend meetings with the parents (6). They can speak or write in support of or on the behalf of the child and his/her parents. The advocate can draft letters and written requests to school and district personnel, as well as complaints to school districts and the SEA (7).

Disability advocates can also provide parents with important information about their child's educational rights and assist them in navigating through negotiations and dispute resolutions with school districts. A special education advocate is not an attorney and should recommend that the family secures a special education attorney if the case goes to mediation or due process (6). Many states have nonprofit advocacy groups that are for children with special needs; the individual practitioner is encouraged to contact his/her state's web site or a social worker to help find what specific state-level resources are available.

LEGAL REPRESENTATION

Despite attempts at solving conflicts with schools, parents must sometimes resort to attaining legal representation through a special education attorney. An attorney that specializes in special education can guide parents through the process of filing for a due process hearing and can represent them at the hearing and possible appeals (8).

SUMMARY

The vast majority of children are beautifully served in this country's educational system. Indeed, national, state, and local educational systems do an incredible amount of outstanding assessment and services for children and teenagers whose widely different autistic spectrum disorder diagnoses require an exceptional sensitivity and creative solutions. In rare situations, if a child's needs are not being met adequately, the primary care physician (PCP) can be instrumental in guiding parents on how to best access services through public schools. Parents can be overwhelmed with what seems like an overwhelming process; however, it behooves all involved to maintain a spirit of mutual cooperation and good will. Tempting as it may be for some situations to escalate to an adversarial or combative situation, such stances rarely yield the positive outcome that is best for the child. Encouragement from the PCP to have families remain open, positive, and cooperative can be incredibly helpful.

REFERENCES

1. Wright PW, Wright PD. How to resolve special education disputes: negotiation, mediation & litigation. http://www.wrightslaw.com/info/mediate.negot.disputes.htm. Retrieved July 2, 2010.
2. Public Law 108-446. *Individuals with Disabilities Education Act of 2004* (IDEA), 20 U.S.C. §1400 et seq.
3. Logsdon A. *Special Education Due Process Hearing—Exploring Special Education Hearings.* http://learningdisabilities.about.com. Retrieved July 2, 2010.
4. Association of Family and Conciliation Courts (formerly Academy of Family Mediators). http://www.afccnet.org. Retrieved July 2, 2010.
5. Wright PW, Wright PD. *What Is mediation? How Does It Work?* http://www.wrightslaw.com/advoc/articles/mediation_faq.html. Retrieved July 2, 2010.
6. Education Center. http://www.ed-center.com/special_education_advocate. Retrieved June 23, 2010.
7. Stiff Exkorn K. *The Autism Sourcebook.* NY: Harper Collins; 2005.
8. Frishman SR. *Special advocacy 101.* http://www.iser.com/resources/advocacy-terms.html. Retrieved July 3, 2010.

Resources for Clinicians/ Resources for Families

1. **Helpful Web sites and links**
   a. American Academy of Neurology
      Screening guidelines for clinicians managing autism:
      http://aan.com/professionals/practice/
      guidelines/guideline_summaries/
      Autism_Guideline_for_Clinicians.pdf
      Screening guidelines for parents:
      http://aan.com/professionals/practice/
      guidelines/guideline_summaries/
      Autism_Guideline_for_Patients.pdf
      Global developmental delay:
      Clinical guidelines for clinicians
      http://www.neurology.org/cgi/reprint/60/
      3/367.pdf
      http://aan.com/professionals/practice/
      guidelines/guideline_summaries/Global_
      Devlopmental_Delay_Clinicians.pdf
   b. American Academy of Pediatrics
      Clinical guidelines for autism:
      http://aappolicy.aappublications.org/cgi/
      content/full/pediatrics%3B120/5/1162
   c. American Academy of Child and Adolescent Psychiatry
      Practice parameters for clinicians managing autism:
      http://www.aacap.org/galleries/Practice
      Parameters/Autism.pdf
      Practice parameters for clinicians managing children with mental retardation and comorbid conditions:
      http://www.aacap.org/galleries/Practice
      Parameters/Mr.pdfFor

2. **Books**

Accardo PJ. *Capute & Accardo's Neurodevelopmental Disabilities in Infancy and Childhood: The Spectrum of Neurodevelopmental Disabilities*. 3rd ed. Vol 2. Paul H Brookes Pub Co; 2008.

Rapin I. *Preschool Children with Inadequate Communication. Clinics in Developmental Medicine*. Raven Press; 1996.

Riva D, Rapin I, Zardini G, Libbey J. *Language: Normal and Pathological Development— Hardcover*. Eurotext Ltd; 2006.

Segaolitz SJ, Rapin I. *Handbook of Neuropsychology*. Vol 7. Elsevier Science Ltd; 1994.

Tuchman R, Rapin I. *Autism: A Neurological Disorder of Early Brain Development*. International Child Neurology Association; 2006.

Volkmar F, Paul R, Klin A, Cohen DJ (eds). *Handbook of Autism and Pervasive Developmental Disorders, Assessment, Interventions, and Policy*. 3rd ed. Vol 2. Wiley; 2005.

RESOURCES FOR FAMILIES

1. **Helpful Web sites and links for families**

The Child with Autism. http://www.aacap.org/cs/
root/facts_for_families/the_child_with_autism

Asperger's Disorder. http://www.aacap.org/cs/root/
facts_for_families/aspergers_disorder

Self Injury in Adolescents. http://www.aacap.org/
cs/root/facts_for_families/selfinjury_in_
adolescents

Children Who Are Mentally Retarded.
http://www.aacap.org/cs/root/facts_for_
families/children_who_are_mentally_retarded

Services in School for Children with Special Needs: What Parents Need to Know. http://
www.aacap.org/cs/root/facts_for_families/
services_in_school_for_children_with_
special_needs_what_parents_need_to_know

Psychiatric Medication for Children and Adolescents Part I – How Medications Are Used.
http://www.aacap.org/cs/root/facts_for_
families/psychiatric_medication_for_
children_and_adolescents_part_ihow_
medications_are_used

Where to Find Help for Your Child. http://www.
aacap.org/cs/root/facts_for_families/where_to_
find_help_for_your_child

2. **Books**

Attwood T. *The Complete Guide to Asperger's Syndrome*. 1st ed. Jessica Kingsley Publishers; 2008.

Baker J. *Preparing for Life: The Complete Guide for Transitioning to Adulthood for Those with Autism and Asperger's Syndrome*. 1st ed. Future Horizons; 2006.

Cafiero J. *Meaningful Exchanges for People with Autism: An Introduction to Augmentative & Alternative Communication (Topics in Autism)*. 1st ed. Woodbine House; 2005.

Cassada R. *The Anger Workbook for Teens: Activities to Help You Deal with Anger and Frustration.* Workbook edition. Lohmann Instant Help Books; 2009.

Cooper B. *The Social Success Workbook for Teens: Skill-building Activities for Teens with Nonverbal Learning Disorder, Asperger's Disorder, & Other Social-skill Problems.* 1st ed. New Harbinger Publications; 2008.

Exkorn, KS. T*he Autism Sourcebook: Everything You Need to Know About Diagnosis, Treatment, Coping, and Healing.* 1st ed. William Morrow; 2005.

Grandin T. *The Way I See It: A Personal Look at Autism and Asperger's.* 1st ed. Future Horizons; 2008.

Grandin T. *Thinking in Pictures: My Life with Autism.* Exp Mti edition. Vintage; 2010.

Grandin T. *Emergence: Labeled Autistic.* Warner Books; 1996.

Grandin T. *The Unwritten Rules of Social Relationships: Decoding Social Mysteries Through the Unique Perspectives of Autism.* Horizons; 2005.

Grandin T. *Developing Talents: Careers for Individuals with Asperger Syndrome and High-functioning Autism - Updated, Expanded Edition.* Autism Asperger Publishing Company; 2008.

Klin A, Volkmar FR, Sparrow, SS. *Asperger Syndrome.* 1st ed. Guilford Press; 2000.

Schab LM. *The Anxiety Workbook for Teens: Activities to Help You Deal with Anxiety & Worry.* 1st ed. New Harbinger Publications; 2008.

Schab LM. *Beyond the Blues: A Workbook to Help Teens Overcome Depression.* 1st ed. Instant Help Books; 2008.

Autism Resources

ORGANIZATIONS AND CENTERS

For Parents

Aspergers Disorder
www.aacap.org/cs/root/facts_for_families/
    aspergers_disorder

Autism Society of America (ASA)
www.autism-society.org
    ASA is a national support network for individ-
    uals with autism and their families. Links are
    available on autism, advocacy, public aware-
    ness, research, and educational opportunities.

Autism Speaks
www.autismspeaks.org
    Autism Speaks is an organization dedicated to
    funding global biomedical research into the
    causes, prevention, treatments, and cure for
    autism, and to raising public awareness about
    autism and its effects on individuals, families,
    and society.

Bright Futures
www.brightfutures.aap.org/web/
    A national initiative to promote and improve
    the health and well-being of infants, children,
    and adolescents. The site includes publications,
    training tools, and distance learning materials.

Cambridge Center for Behavioral Studies
www.behavior.org/autism
    The site provides explanation and information
    about ABA therapy.

Children Who Are Mentally Retarded
www.aacap.org/cs/root/facts_for_families/
    children_who_are_mentally_retarded

Families for Effective Autism Treatment
www.feat.org/
    A nonprofit organization of parents and con-
    cerned professionals dedicated to providing
    education, workshops, and support for children
    with autism and their families.

First Signs
www.firstsigns.org
    First Signs is a national nonprofit organization
    dedicated to educating parents and physicians
    about the early warning signs of autism and
    other developmental disorders. The site offers
    information on screening, development,
    referral, treatment, and resources.

Floortime Foundation
www.floortime.org
    The site provides explanation and information
    about Floortime therapy.

Medline Plus—Asperger's Syndrome
www.nlm.nih.gov/medlineplus/
    aspergerssyndrome.html
    A service of the U.S. National Library of
    Medicine and the National Institutes of Health.
    Includes information in Spanish.

Medline Plus—Autism
www.nlm.nih.gov/medlineplus/autism.html
    A service of the U.S. National Library of
    Medicine and the National Institutes of Health.
    Includes information in Spanish.

Online Asperger Syndrome and Support (OASIS)
www.udel.edu/bkirby/asperger
    OASIS provides information and support on
    Asperger's syndrome.

Psychiatric Medication for Children and
    Adolescents Part I – How Medications
    Are Used
www.aacap.org/cs/root/facts_for_families/
    psychiatric_medication_for_children_and_
    adolescents_part_ihow_medications_are_used

Self-Injury in Adolescents
www.aacap.org/cs/root/facts_for_families/
    selfinjury_in_adolescents

Services in School for Children with Special
    Needs: What Parents Need to Know
www.aacap.org/cs/root/facts_for_families/
    services_in_school_for_children_with_
    special_needs_what_parents_need_to_know

TEACCH
www.teacch.com
    The site provides explanation and information
    about the TEACCH program.

The Child with Autism
www.aacap.org/cs/root/facts_for_families/the_
    child_with_autism

Where to Find Help for Your Child
www.aacap.org/cs/root/facts_for_families/
    where_to_find_help_for_your_child

Zero to Three
www.zerotothree.org
    This site includes resources for parents and
    professionals.

For Clinicians

American Academy of Child and Adolescent Psychiatry
Practice parameters for clinicians managing autism:
http://www.aacap.org/galleries/PracticeParameters/Autism.pdf
and
Practice parameters for clinicians managing children with mental retardation and comorbid conditions:
http://www.aacap.org/galleries/PracticeParameters/Mr.pdfFor
American Academy of Pediatrics (AAP)
www.aap.org
   The site lists resources that include books and articles, and provides articles on current topics.
Clinical guidelines for autism:
aappolicy.aappublications.org/cgi/content/full/pediatrics%3B120/5/1162
American Academy of Family Physicians (AAFP)
www.aafp.org
American Academy of Neurology
Autism:
Screening guidelines for clinicians:
aan.com/professionals/practice/guidelines/guideline_summaries/Autism_Guideline_for_Clinicians.pdf
Screening guidelines for parents:
aan.com/professionals/practice/guidelines/guideline_summaries/Autism_Guideline_for_Patients.pdf
Global delay:
Clinical guidelines for clinicians:
www.neurology.org/cgi/reprint/60/3/367.pdf
and
aan.com/professionals/practice/guidelines/guideline_summaries/Global_Devlopmental_Delay_Clinicians.pdf
Autism Information Center
cdc.gov/ncbddd/dd/ddautism.htm
National Center on Birth Defects and Developmental Disabilities
Autism Research Institute (ARI)
www.autism.com/ari/
   Conducts research on the causes of autism and on the methods of preventing, diagnosing, and treating autism and other severe behavioral disorders of childhood.

FEDERAL/NATIONAL ORGANIZATIONS

Child Find (component of IDEA)
www.childfindidea.org
   Child Find is a part of IDEA and provides information related to the early identification of young children and their families who may benefit from early intervention or education services.
Department of Education (DOE)
www.ed.gov/index.jsp
   The DOE provides information related to early childhood education and assessing development in children.
Individuals with Disabilities Education Act (IDEA)
www.nectac.org/idea/idea.asp
   The National Early Childhood Technical Assistance Center Web site provides the full text of the IDEA legislation and other related information.
National Center on Birth Defects and Developmental Disabilities (NCBDDD)
www.cdc.gov/ncbddd/
   NCBDDD is a part of the Centers for Disease Control and Prevention (CDC) and promotes the health of babies, children, and adults to enhance the potential for full, productive living.
National Institute on Mental Health (NIMH)
http://www.nimh.nih.gov/publicat/autism.cfm
   The National Institute on Mental Health: Autism is an online autism publication, including a definition of autism and information on national resources and supports.

LEGAL/ADVOCACY ORGANIZATIONS AND INFORMATION

Family Education Network
www.familyeducation.com
   This site provides a great expanse of information to parents generally, and includes a number of articles written by a special education attorney for parents of children with disabilities and their advocates regarding the special education system.
Special Education Advocate (Wrights Law)
www.wrightslaw.com
   This site provides legal information about special education law and advocacy for students with disabilities.
Special Education Law (Reed Martin)
www.reedmartin.com
   This site provides informational resource for parents and school personnel advocating for children with special needs.

INFORMATION IN SPANISH

Asociacion Nuevo Horizonte
www.autismo.com/
    Directorio de recursos relacionados con el
    autismo, articulos, congresos, y tablon de
    mensajes.
Autismo
www.autisme.com/

Definicion, tratamientos, biblografia, y organizaciones en Espana.

DISCLAIMER: Links to these sites are included for information only. Reference to any treatment, therapy option, product or to any program, service, treatment, or product provider is not an endorsement of the authors.

Behavior-Based Handouts

HEADBANGING

Granana N, Tuchman RF, Painter MJ. A child with severe head banging. *Semin Pediatr Neurol.* 1999;6(3):221–224.

How to Control Head-Banging Sleep Disorders. http://www.ehowcom/how_4840158_control-headbanging-sleep-disorders.html

Understanding and Treating Self-Injurious Behavior. http://www.autism.com/ind_self-injurious_behavior_treat.asp

SLEEPLESSNESS

Establishing Positive Sleep Patterns for Children on the Autism Spectrum. http://www.autism-society.org/site/DocServer/LWA_Sleep.pdf?docID=4184

Helping Your Child with Autism Get a Good Night's Sleep. http://www.webmdcom/brain/autism/helping-your-child-with-autism-get-a-good-nights-sleep

Durand MV. *Sleep Better! A Guide to Improving Sleep for Children with Special Needs.* Paul H Brookes Publishing Co; 1998.

Richdale AL. Sleep problems in autism: prevalence, cause, and intervention. *Dev Med Child Neurol.* 1999;41:60–66.

Wiggs L, Stores G. Sleep patterns and sleep disorders in children with autistic spectrum disorders: insights using parent report and actigraphy. *Dev Med Child Neurol.* 2004;46: 372–380.

Williams PG, Sears LL, Allard A. Sleep problems in children with autism. *J Sleep Res.* 2004;13: 265–268.

AGGRESSION

Hartley SL, Sikora DM, McCoy R. Prevalence and risk factors of maladaptive behavior in young children with autistic disorder. *J Intellect Disabil Res.* 2008;52(10):819–829.

Parikh MS, Kolevzon A, Hollander E. Psychopharmacology of aggression in children and adolescents with autism: a critical review of efficacy and tolerability *J Child Adolesc Psychopharmacol.* 2008;18(2):157–178.

Pediatric Psychopharmacology. American Psychiatric Association, 2008. http://www.psych.org/MainMenu/EducationCareerDevelopment/LifeLongLearning/AnnualMeetingOnline/PediatricPsychopharmacology.aspx

Treatment of Aggression: Aggression and Autism Impulsivity. http://cme.medscape.com/viewarticle/420328

SEXUAL INAPPROPRIATENESS

Koller R. Sexuality and adolescents with autism. *Sex Dis.* 2000;18(2):125–135. http://www.thefate.org/library/public_document/Adaptive%20Life%20Skills-/Sex%20Education/Autism%20and%20Sexuality.pdf

Realmuto GM, Ruble LA. Sexual behaviors in autism: problems of definition and management. *J Autism Dev Disord.* 1999;29(2): 121–127.

Social/Sexual Awareness for Persons with Disabilities. http://www.autism.com/ind_social_sexual_awareness.asp

TANTRUMS

Behavior Modification: Temper Tantrums. http://www.childbrain.com/pddq11.shtml

Scahill L, Koenig K, Carroll DH, Pachler M. Risperidone approved for the treatment of serious behavioral problems in children with autism. *J Child Adolesc Psychiatr Nurs.* 2007. http://findarticlescom/p/articles/mi_qa3892/is_200708/ai_n19512001/

Shea S, Turgay A, Carroll A, et al. Risperidone in the treatment of disruptive behavioral symptoms in children with autistic or other pervasive developmental disorders. *Pediatrics.* 2004;114(5):e634–e641.

Whitaker P, Joy H, Edwards D, Harley J. *Challenging Behavior and Autism: Making Sense—Making Progress; a Guide to Preventing and Managing Challenging Behavior for Parents and Teachers.* National Autistic Society; 2001.

School Interactions

PARENT HANDOUT FOR ATTENDING A CHILD'S ARD/IEP MEETING

Using the ARD/IEP Agenda to Understand the Special Education Process. http://www.texasprojectfirst.org/ARDIEP.html

How to Survive an ARD Meeting. http://www.ehow.com/how_2164328_survive-ard-meeting.html

Admission, Review and Dismissal Committee Meetings (ARDs). http://www.atpe.org/protection/YourStudentsAndParents/ards.asp

IEP Meeting Preparation. http://www.humboldtcasa.org/Chapter%2010%20IEP%20Meeting%20Preparation.pdf

PARENT QUESTIONNAIRE FOR SCHOOL

Six Questions Parents Should Ask at an ARD Meeting. http://lifeplanseminar.com/uploads/Six_Questions_Parents_Should_Ask_at_an_ARD_Meeting.pdf

IEP Meeting Preparation Checklist for Parents. http://www.arcfc.org/documents/IEPChecklist2007.pdf

SAMPLE LETTER FROM PARENT/GUARDIAN TO SCHOOL

Sample School Letter from Parent/Guardian

Date

Name of Special Education Director
Director of Special Education
School System Name
Street Address
City, State, Zip Code

Dear Ms./Mr. (Name of Special Education Director)

    I am requesting an individual comprehensive evaluation for my child, (Child's Name), to determine if he/she is eligible for special education services. He/She is in (Grade Level) at (School Name). His/Her date of birth is (Birth Date). (Child's name) has been struggling with _____ (reading, writing, math, attention, social skills, and/or behavior) since ____ (e.g., grade, age). He/She has been identified as having (name of disability) by (name of professional). I've enclosed a copy of the report(s).

    I would like to meet with the special education chairperson for my child's school before testing begins so that I might share information and discuss the evaluation procedures, as well as sign the written permission document to allow the assessment of my child. I would like a copy of the written report from each evaluator so that I can review them before meeting to discuss the evaluation results.

    We have tried the following to help (child's name):

    [Parents should include in this section strategies employed at home, tutors (it should be noted if these services have been paid out of pocket), as well as accommodations/modifications reported by teachers (documentation such as parent/teacher conference notes or e-mails are important). District or state assessment results that indicate below grade-level performance or failure to meet criteria, report cards, progress reports, or samples of work that document the child's struggles should also be included.]

    In keeping with *Individuals with Disabilities Education Act* (IDEA) requirement, I understand that I should receive communication from you within 10 days of receipt of this letter. I look forward to working with you, for the benefit of my child's education.

Sincerely,

Name
Address
Phone number

cc: *the child's principal (if letter is addressed to another administrator) and the child's teacher*

SAMPLE MEDICAL LETTERS OF NECESSITY FROM PCP TO SCHOOL

Date

To Whom It May Concern

I am the pediatrician for (child's name) and have cared for him/her for the past _____ years. (Child's name) has been diagnosed with _____ and requires special education or Section 504 services in order for him/her to have equitable access to an appropriate and purposeful education.

Symptoms of his/her disorder/illness include _____. He/she is prescribed _____ to assist him; however, the medication does not ameliorate his symptoms. His/her performance, attention, energy, alertness, etc., would be expected to be variable on a day-to-day basis or during different times of the day.

I welcome the opportunity to discuss "Patient's" situation further with you if needed and hope you will support these necessary medical services.

Thank you in advance for your assistance in this matter.

Sincerely,

Name
Contact information

PRESCRIPTION PAD REQUEST FROM PCP TO SCHOOL

An alternative to a letter or as an initial request for services, a diagnosis and request for services can be made on a script pad, such as

(Child's name) qualifies under the autism spectrum, most likely PDD-NOS.

Please enroll him/her in the special education program at his/her school.

or

(Child's name) has been diagnosed with a global developmental delay.

Please provide him/her with the appropriate educational and intervention services.

KEY WORDS

Autism
Autism spectrum disorders
Asperger syndrome
Cognitive deficit
Fragile X syndrome
Neuropathologic abnormalities
Pervasive developmental disorders
Self-injurious behaviors

ABBREVIATIONS

AAC—alternative augmentative communication
ABC—Autism behavior checklist
AAN –American Academy of Neurology
AAP—American Academy of Pediatrics
AD—autistic disorder
ADA—Americans with Disabilities Act
ADHD—attention-deficit/hyperactivity disorder
ADI—autism diagnostic interview
ADOS—autism diagnostic observation schedule
APE—adaptive physical education
ARD—admission, review, and dismissal
AS—Asperger syndrome
ASD—autism spectrum disorder
ASDS—Asperger syndrome diagnostic scale
AT—assistive technology
AU—autism
BD—behavior disorder
BIP—behavior intervention plan
CA—chronological age
CARS—childhood autism rating scale
CAST—childhood Asperger syndrome test
CHAT—checklist for autism in toddlers
DSM—*Diagnostic and Statistical Manual of Mental Disorders*
ED—emotionally disturbed
EEG—electroencephalography
EI—early intervention
ESY—extended school year
FAPE—free appropriate public education
FAS—fetal alcohol syndrome

FBA—functional behavior assessment
FERPA—Family Education Rights and Privacy Act
FIE—full individual evaluation
FISH—fluorescence in situ hybridization
FXS—fragile X syndrome
GARS—Gilliam autism rating scale
GDD—global developmental delay
IDEA—Individuals with Disabilities Education Act
IEE—individual education evaluation
IEP—individual education plan
K-ABC—Kaufman assessment battery for children
LD—learning disability
LRI—least restrictive environment
M-CHAT—modified checklist for autism in toddlers
MPH—methylphenidate
MR—mental retardation
MMR—measles-mumps–rubella
MSEL—Mullen scales of early learning
NCLB—no child left behind
OCD—obsessive–compulsive disorder
ODD—oppositional defiant disorder
OHI—other health impaired
PDD-NOS—pervasive developmental disorder—not otherwise specified
PCP—primary care practitioner
PEP—psychoeducational profile test
SI—sensory integration
SSRI—selective serotonin reuptake inhibitor
TCA—tricyclic antidepressant
TPL—test of pragmatic language
VABS—Vineland adaptive behavior scales
WPPSI—Wechsler preschool and primary scale of intelligence
WAIS—Wechsler adult intelligence scale
WIAT—Wechsler individual achievement test
WISC—Wechsler intelligence test for children
WJ—Woodcock–Johnson: tests of cognitive abilities and tests of achievement

BIBLIOGRAPHY

Doyle BT, Lland ED. *Los Trastornos del Espectro de Autismo de la A a la Z* (Autism Disorders from A to Z). Emily Lland, Inc; 2005.

Exkorn KS. *The Autism Sourcebook: Everything You Need to Know About Diagnosis, Treatment, Coping, and Healing.* 1st ed. William Morrow; 2005.

Howlin P. *Autism and Asperger Syndrome: Preparing for Adulthood.* Routledge; 2004.

Grandin T. *The Way I See It: A Personal Look at Autism and Asperger's.* Future Horizons, Inc, 2008. Temple provides helpful do's and don'ts, practical strategies, and try-it-now tips, all based on her "insider" perspective and a great deal of research.

Grandin T. *Thinking in Pictures: My Life with Autism.* Exp Mti edition. Vintage; 2010.

Grandin T. *Emergence: Labeled Autistic.* Warner Books; 1996.

Grandin T. *The Unwritten Rules of Social Relationships: Decoding Social Mysteries Through the Unique Perspectives of Autism.* Horizons; 2005.

Grandin T. *Developing Talents: Careers for Individuals with Asperger Syndrome and High-functioning Autism - Updated.* Expanded Edition. Autism Asperger Publishing Company; 2008.

For Parents and Teachers

Attwood T. *The Complete Guide to Asperger's Syndrome.* Jessica Kinglsey Publishing; 2008.

Bareket R. *Playing It Right! Social Skills Activities for Parents and Teachers of Young Children with Autism Spectrum Disorders Including Asperger Syndrome and Autism.* Autism Asperger Publishing Co; 2006.

Collins AW, Collins S. *Autism: Now What? The Primer of Parents.* Phat Art 4; 2002.

Fouse B, Wheeler M. *A Treasure Chest of Behavioral Strategies for Individuals with Autism.* Future Horizons; 1997.

Notbohm E, Zysk V. *1001 Great Ideas of Teaching and Raising Children with Autism Spectrum Disorders.* 2nd ed. Future Horizons, Inc; 2010.

Satkiewicz-Gayhardt V, Peerenboom B, Campbell R. *Crossing Bridges: A Parent's Perspective on Coping After a Child Is Diagnosed with Autism/PDD.* Autism Society of New Hampshire; 2007.

Siegel B, Silverstein S. *What About Me? Growing up with a Developmentally Disabled Sibling.* Perseus Publishing; 1995.

Wheeler M. *Toilet Training for Individuals with Autism or Other Developmental Issues.* Future Horizons, Inc; 2007.

Wiseman ND. *The First Year-Autism Spectrum Disorders: An Essential Guide for the Newly Diagnosed Child.* Da Capo Press; 2009.

For Clinicians

Accardo PJ. *Capute & Accardo's Neurodevelopmental Disabilities in Infancy and Childhood: The Spectrum of Neurodevelopmental Disabilities.* 3rd ed. Vol 2. Paul H Brookes Pub Co; 2008.

Klin A, Volkmar FR, Sparrow, SS. *Asperger Syndrome.* Guilford Press; 2000.

Rapin I. *Preschool Children with Inadequate Communication (Clinics in Developmental Medicine).* Raven Press; 1996.

Riva D, Rapin I, Zardini G, Libbey J. *Language: Normal and Pathological Development – Hardcover.* Eurotext Ltd; 2006.

Segaolitz SJ, Rapin I. *Handbook of Neuropsychology.* Vol 7. Elsevier Science Ltd; 1994.

Tuchman R, Rapin I. *Autism: A Neurological Disorder of Early Brain Development.* International Child Neurology Association; 2006.

Volkmar F, Paul R, Klin A, Cohen DJ (eds). *Handbook of Autism and Pervasive Developmental Disorders, Assessment, Interventions, and Policy.* 3rd ed. Vol 2. Wiley; 2005.

For Individuals with ASD

Baker J. *Preparing for Life: The Complete Guide for Transitioning to Adulthood for Those with Autism and Asperger's Syndrome.* 1st ed. Future Horizons; 2006.

Cafiero J. *Meaningful Exchanges for People with Autism: An Introduction to Augmentative & Alternative Communication (Topics in Autism).* 1st ed. Woodbine House; 2005.

Cassada R. *The Anger Workbook for Teens: Activities to Help You Deal with Anger and Frustration.* Workbook edition. Lohmann Instant Help Books; 2009.

Cooper B. *The Social Success Workbook for Teens: Skill-building Activities for Teens with Nonverbal Learning Disorder, Asperger's Disorder, & Other Social-skill Problems.* 1st ed. New Harbinger Publications; 2008.

Schab LM. *The Anxiety Workbook for Teens: Activities to Help You Deal with Anxiety & Worry.* 1st ed. New Harbinger Publications; 2008.

Schab LM. *Beyond the Blues: A Workbook to Help Teens Overcome Depression.* 1st ed. Instant Help Books; 2008.

For Siblings

Beach F. *Everybody Is Different: A Book for Young People Who Have Brothers or Sisters with Autism, for Ages 8–16.* The National Autistic Society; 2001.

Harris S. *Siblings of Children with Autism: A Guide for Families.* 2nd ed. Woodbine Press; 2003.

Peralta S. *All About My Brother: Written by 8-Year-Old Sarah, Sister of a Nonverbal Younger Brother with Autism. For Children Ages 6–10.* Autism Asperger Publishing Company; 2002.

Sullivan C. *I Love My Brother. A Picture Book Written by 4-Year-Old Connor About His 2-Year-Old Brother Sean, Who Has Autism. For Preschool and Kindergarten Children.* Phat Art 4 Publishing; 2001.

For Classmates/Peers

Bishop B. *My Friend with Autism.* Arlington, TX: Future Horizons; 2002. Offers elementary-age classmates concrete ways to develop friendships with children with autism, for ages 4–10.

Ellis M. *Keisha's Doors* (English and Spanish versions), part I of a series. Speech Kids Texas Press; 2005. For ages 4 through 8.

Online Book Resources

Children's Disability Information. www.childrensdisabilities.info/parenting/spec-books.html

Future Horizons. www.futurehorizons-autism.com/

Jessica Kingsley Publishers. www.jkp.com/

Speech Kids Texas Press. http://www.speechkidstexaspress.com/

Woodbine House. www.woodbinehouse.com/

DISCLAIMER: Links to these sites are included for information only. Reference to any treatment, therapy option, product or to any program, service, treatment, or product provider is not an endorsement of the authors.

INDEX

Note: Page numbers followed by t indicate tables.